Cocaine and Methamphetamine Dependence

Advances in Treatment

Cocaine and Methamphetamine Dependence
Advances in Treatment

Edited by

Thomas R. Kosten, M.D.
Thomas F. Newton, M.D.
Richard De La Garza II, Ph.D.
Colin N. Haile, M.D., Ph.D.

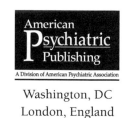

American Psychiatric Publishing
A Division of American Psychiatric Association

Washington, DC
London, England

Copyright © 2012 American Psychiatric Association
ALL RIGHTS RESERVED
Manufactured in the United States of America on acid-free paper
15   14   13   12   11   5   4   3   2   1
First Edition
Typeset in Helvetica and Berkeley

American Psychiatric Publishing
A Division of American Psychiatric Association
1000 Wilson Boulevard
Arlington, VA 22209-3901
www.appi.org

Library of Congress Cataloging-in-Publication Data
Cocaine and methamphetamine dependence : advances in treatment / edited by Thomas R. Kosten ... [et al.]. — 1st ed.
    p. ; cm.
Includes bibliographical references and index.
ISBN 978-1-58562-407-2 (pbk. : alk. paper)
I. Kosten, Thomas R.
[DNLM: 1. Cocaine-Related Disorders—therapy. 2. Amphetamine-Related Disorders—therapy. 3. Behavior Therapy. 4. Psychotropic Drugs—therapeutic use. WM 280]
LC classification not assigned
615.7'88—dc23

                                                                2011025966
British Library Cataloguing in Publication Data
A CIP record is available from the British Library.

Contents

Contributors

Richard De La Garza II, Ph.D.
Associate Professor of Psychiatry, Neuroscience, and Pharmacology, Baylor College of Medicine and Michael E. DeBakey Veterans Affairs (VA) Medical Center; Research Director and Associate Professor, Departments of Psychiatric Oncology and Behavioral Science, University of Texas M.D. Anderson Cancer Center, Houston, Texas

Carrie L. Dodrill, Ph.D.
Psychologist, Michael E. DeBakey VA Medical Center, Houston, Texas

Rachel Fintzy, M.A.
Project Director, UCLA Integrated Substance Abuse Programs, David Geffen School of Medicine, University of California, Los Angeles

Valerie A. Gruber, Ph.D., M.P.H.
Clinical Professor, Department of Psychiatry, University of California, San Francisco

Colin N. Haile, M.D., Ph.D.
Assistant Professor, Menninger Department of Psychiatry and Behavioral Sciences, Baylor College of Medicine and Michael E. DeBakey VA Medical Center, Houston, Texas

Ari D. Kalechstein, Ph.D.
Adjunct Associate Professor, Menninger Department of Psychiatry and Behavioral Sciences, Baylor College of Medicine and Michael E DeBakey VA Medical Center, Houston, Texas

Herbert D. Kleber, M.D.
Professor, Department of Psychiatry, Columbia University, and Director, Division of Substance Abuse, New York State Psychiatric Institute, New York, New York

Thomas R. Kosten, M.D.
J.H. Waggoner Chair and Professor of Psychiatry, Pharmacology and Neuro-science, Baylor College of Medicine; Professor of Psychiatry and Epidemiology, M.D. Anderson Cancer Center; and Director, VA National Substance Use Disorders Quality Enhancement Research Initiative (QUERI), Houston, Texas

Elinore F. McCance-Katz, M.D., Ph.D.
Professor, Department of Psychiatry, University of California, San Francisco

Thomas F. Newton, M.D.
Professor, Menninger Department of Psychiatry and Behavioral Sciences and Department of Pharmacology, Baylor College of Medicine and Michael E. DeBakey VA Medical Center, Houston, Texas

Jin H. Yoon, Ph.D.
Assistant Professor, Menninger Department of Psychiatry and Behavioral Sciences, Baylor College of Medicine, Houston, Texas

Foreword

This book provides a comprehensive summary of what a clinician needs to know about stimulant dependence and its treatment in order to move beyond the basics of this complex disorder as presented in *The American Psychiatric Publishing Textbook of Substance Abuse Treatment* (Galanter and Kleber 2008). The textbook covers the material that a general psychiatrist or primary care physician needs for appropriate referral and initial management of patients with these complex disorders, for which no U.S. Food and Drug Administration (FDA)–approved pharmacotherapies yet exist, but treatments for these disorders are evolving rapidly. The present volume more closely examines stimulant abuse and its changing epidemiologies and treatment models.

As outlined in Chapter 1 of this volume, cocaine, methamphetamine (METH), and amphetamine (AMPH) abuse and dependence differ substantially in geographic distribution among North American cities and rural areas, as well as in Europe and Asia. The Philippines have the world's highest rates of AMPH abuse, with estimates that over 2.9% of the population are abusers (Ahmad 2003).

The criminal justice responses to these stimulant epidemics have produced some enlightened and humane linkages between the criminal justice system and treatment, such as "drug courts," where judges order legally supervised treatment for stimulant abusers rather than sending them to prison. Treatment has also been introduced into the prisons themselves and includes options for reducing the duration of imprisonment through work-release programs. These legal innovations are critical for the estimated 1.6 million current (on any given day) cocaine abusers and 502,000 current METH abusers (2009 estimates; Substance Abuse and Mental Health Services Administration 2010b). Another intervention initiated by the criminal justice system rapidly reduced small clandestine METH laboratories from more than 16,000 in 2004 to about 5,000 by 2007 as law enforcement efforts to control supplies of the ephedrine precursors and to find and destroy these laboratories were effective. These efforts increased the price of METH by over 80% while its purity decreased by 26%, and the indicators in almost all metropolitan areas showed stable or reduced METH use (although there appeared to be somewhat of a rebound in METH availability during 2008).

Despite such efforts, there is still a steady number of new users and casualties from stimulant use: the 30-day prevalence of cocaine abuse among eighth, tenth, and twelfth graders increased more than twofold between 1991 and 1998 and recently increased again in 2009 and 2010 (Johnston et al. 2010).

Overall, cocaine dependence complications are common, being involved in one of every three drug-related emergency department visits, and cocaine has substantial social and economic impacts on those afflicted (McLellan et al. 2000; Substance Abuse and Mental Health Services Administration 2010b). Moreover, from 2007 through 2009, the United States had 2.5 million cocaine abusers using regularly, and in 2007 only 809,000 of them received treatment (Substance Abuse and Mental Health Services Administration 2010c). Coroners' reports (Graham and Hanzlick 2008; Kaye et al. 2008) relate stimulants to the direct cause of death in 25% of cocaine overdoses and 68% of METH overdoses, or identify stimulant use as an antecedent of cardiovascular or other medical problems, leading to death, in another 20% of these abusers.

The epidemiology of stimulant abuse is changing because of the increase in pharmaceutical abuse attributable to several factors: 1) increasing numbers of prescriptions have led to greater availability; 2) attention to this form of abuse by the media and in advertising on television and newspapers has stimulated adolescents' interest in it; 3) easy access through family and friends has made this type of abuse cheap and attractive; and 4) lack of proper monitoring of adolescents and of disappearance of drugs in the home or elsewhere has led to underrecognition of addiction (Substance Abuse and Mental Health Services Administration 2010a).

Cocaine and METH abuse and dependence frequently co-occur with other major (i.e., Axis I) mental illnesses, especially schizophrenia, major depression (Hughes et al. 1986), and posttraumatic stress disorder (PTSD) (Jacobsen et al. 2001). Many types of drug use are more common among patients with mental illnesses than among the general population. Patients with mood and anxiety disorders are at less risk for smoking and perhaps for stimulant abuse than patients with schizophrenia, but patients with any of these comorbid disorders smoke at higher rates than control subjects, and many biological and social factors are involved. Psychotic symptoms secondary to METH abuse may not abate after the METH use has stopped and may be associated with heavy alcohol use.

Chapter 2, on the complex pharmacology of stimulants, is outstanding, although not readily summarized in a brief Foreword.

Chapter 3, on symptoms and diagnosis, introduces the plan for DSM-5 to drop the distinction between abuse and dependence, which is a useful change in considering stimulants. In addressing teenage drug use information reports, the author emphasizes the limitations of self-reports; even if anonymous or confidential, they can lead to underreporting because respondents will still give socially acceptable but untruthful answers, such as "I don't" use drugs. A recent study in teens found that hair specimens were 52 times more likely to identify cocaine use compared with self-report. Furthermore, parent hair analyses for cocaine use were 6.5 times more likely to indicate drug use than was parental self-report (Delaney-Black et al. 2010). The SBIRT (Screening, Brief Intervention, and Referral to Treatment), a national program for screening and brief interventions with drug abusers, indicates that such urine screening in emergency departments has particularly high yields for detection and for reductions in health care utilization with even a single 10- to 15-minute intervention focused on the substance abuse.

Subjective and behavioral responses to stimulants, including both tolerance of and sensitization to behavioral effects, are also detailed in Chapter 3. Sensitization for AMPH-induced psychosis may persist despite long periods of abstinence and may be characterized by delusions, paranoid thinking, and stereotyped compulsive behavior. Dependence and withdrawal syndromes are reviewed, and treatments for the range of stimulant complications are considered (Gay 1982).

A comprehensive assessment of the patient involves the management of aberrant behaviors such as intoxication, violence, suicidality, impaired cognitive functioning, and uncontrolled affective displays. Suicidal ideation may be intense but may clear within hours. In the case of intoxication, blood and urine tests can help to determine the relevant stimulant(s) involved, as well as to identify withdrawal from another drug that is masked or exacerbated by concurrent stimulant dependence. Differences in developmental, gender, and cultural presentations in the natural history of stimulant dependence are also considered in Chapter 3.

The differential diagnosis of stimulant-induced intoxication and withdrawal can require distinguishing these from a wide range of psychiatric disorders, and up to a month of abstinence may be required for clear distinctions to be made. However, the introduction of pharmacological treatments, such as antidepressants, does not require such a lengthy delay. Thus, therapeutic and diagnostic distinctions may require different time frames during evaluations of the patient. For example, the symptoms of stimulant withdrawal frequently overlap with those of depressive disorders, and this diagnosis can be particularly difficult to distinguish from protracted withdrawal, which can include sleep and appetite disturbance as well as dysphoria that mimics affective disorders. A clinical vignette addresses whether a patient with stimulant dependence in remission with a confirmed diagnosis of residual attention deficit disorder should be given a trial of methylphenidate.

Chapter 3 closes with a review of biomarkers for stimulant, and particularly cocaine, dependence. These biomarkers include abnormalities in neurotransmitter receptors and transporters that have been noted in animal models and confirmed in human neuroimaging studies of both the dopamine (DA) and serotonin (5-HT) neurotransmitter systems (Volkow et al. 1990), although none of these neuroimaging, neurohormone, or genetic biomarkers have entered general clinical use.

Later chapters focus on treatment and emphasize that the most important component of stimulant treatment involves behavioral therapies, often in combination with adjunctive medications (see Chapters 4 and 5). Although no medications have been FDA approved for use in stimulant dependence, a range of candidate medications, with varying mechanisms of action, have shown some efficacy. Distinguishing among the effectiveness of available behavioral treatments based on outcome has been difficult. A large multisite study showed little difference between drug counseling and two more intensive behavioral therapies, cognitive and supportive-expressive; however, these therapies retain patients in treatment and can lead to abstinence (Crits-Christoph et al. 1999). Overall, these therapies form the platform for any pharmacotherapy in order to engage the patient and facilitate more long-term changes, including prevention of relapse (Carroll 1997; Carroll et al. 2000).

Contingency management (CM) procedures are given significant attention in this book. The authors emphasize that effective CM requires treatment providers to identify an appropriate target as well as a method for assessing the occurrence of the target behavior. Additionally, treatment providers must choose appropriate and effective reinforcers and decide the optimal way to deliver those reinforcers. Positive contingencies have been used to initiate abstinence and prevent relapse, and this approach has been quite successful for managing individuals who abuse cocaine or AMPH (Higgins et al. 1994b, 2000a, 2000b; Petry 2005; Silverman et al. 1996; Weinstock et al. 2007). The goal of this approach has been to decrease behavior maintained by drug reinforcers and increase behavior maintained by nondrug reinforcers by presenting rewards contingent on documented drug abstinence (positive contingencies) and withdrawing privileges contingent on documented drug use (negative contingencies).

Studies illustrate how positive CM procedures facilitate initial abstinence in cocaine-dependent persons. In a 24-week study (Higgins et al. 1994a), cocaine-dependent individuals were randomly assigned to receive either behavioral treatment without incentives or behavioral treatment with incentives (i.e., vouchers exchangeable for goods and services) during weeks 1–12. Then, during weeks 13–24, clients in both groups received a $1.00 lottery ticket for every drug-free urine sample, in addition to behavioral treatment. The group that received the incentives showed significantly greater treatment retention and longer duration of continuous abstinence than the group not receiving the incentives. In a 12-week clinical trial among methadone-maintained cocaine abusers (Silverman et al. 1996), the CM group also achieved significantly longer duration of sustained cocaine abstinence than control subjects. Overall, these findings suggest that incentives contingent on drug abstinence can be a powerful intervention tool for facilitating cocaine abstinence in cocaine- and methadone-maintained cocaine abusers.

Recent studies have further reinforced that abstinence-based incentive procedures are efficacious in improving retention and associated abstinence outcomes in substance abusers. CM interventions implemented in community-based settings, for example, have been successful in improving retention and associated abstinence outcomes (Petry 2005). Combining CM with pharmacotherapies such as bupropion may significantly improve treatment outcomes for cocaine addiction as well (Poling et al. 2006). There is, however, a significantly higher cost associated with the incentives group versus usual-care group (Olmstead et al. 2010). In order to determine the cost-effectiveness of implementing CM to improve patient outcomes in real-world situations, researchers need to determine threshold values for patient outcomes in substance abuse treatment.

As discussed in Chapter 4, cognitive-behavioral therapy (CBT) is also an efficacious intervention for the treatment of stimulant abuse. CBT for stimulant abuse includes functional analyses to determine the client's historical and current triggers for drug use, along with skills training in the management of drug cravings, effective drug-refusal techniques, and general problem-solving and decision-making strategies. Computerized delivery of CBT may effectively address issues commonly associated with regular in-person therapy sessions, such as scarcity of qualified mental health professionals in less populated regions, scheduling problems, transportation issues, and financial constraints.

In a recent pilot study, CBT was examined in conjunction with pharmacotherapy to evaluate length of treatment, drug-free urinalyses, and reduction of alcohol and cocaine craving. Although subjects who received CBT remained in treatment longer than subjects who received CBT and either disulfiram or naltrexone, the combination treatment groups achieved significantly greater reductions in cocaine-positive urinalyses (Grassi et al. 2007). In a study comparing CBT with CM, CM was found to be efficacious during treatment application. While CM may be useful in engaging substance users, retaining them in treatment, and helping them achieve abstinence, CBT has comparable longer-term outcomes (Rawson et al. 2006). Results of previous research also suggest that cognitive deficits predict low retention in outpatient CBT treatment programs for cocaine dependence (Aharonovich et al. 2003, 2006). Future studies should examine the potential impact of differences in cognitive functioning on treatment outcomes and should test group counseling approaches, which offer various assumptions and models to match the needs of specific individuals.

The complex pharmacology and pharmacodynamics of cocaine's action, from the molecular to the behavioral level, is described in Chapter 5 as a foundation for a review of current pharmacotherapies (see also Chapter 2 for a discussion of basic neuropharmacology of stimulants). A key concept for acute reinforcement and euphoria is that different forms of cocaine and AMPH differ in their addictive potency based on how quickly the drug traverses the blood-brain barrier and affects key limbic circuits. Chronic stimulant abuse induces aberrant synaptic plasticity on brain circuits linked to reward learning as well as on other brain circuits. Specifically, cocaine-dependent individuals have decreased DA synthesis, reduced endogenous DA levels, blunted stimulant-induced DA release, reduced D_2/D_3 receptor availability, and increased DA transporter and cortical norepinephrine (NE) transporter levels. These abnormalities have been shown in human neuroimaging studies of limbic brain areas related to DA neurotransmission. Furthermore, vulnerable phenotypes prone to develop cocaine dependence are being noted in both neuroimaging and genetic studies. These abnormalities are defining the brain disease substrate of cocaine dependence and helping researchers to identify appropriate targets for treatment. Newer clinical studies have switched their focus from DA to the NE and glutamate (GLU) neurotransmitter systems in order to develop new pharmacotherapies. A substantial number of clinical trials have identified compounds that theoretically may correct deficiencies in neural circuits and attenuate the reinforcing effects of cocaine in cocaine-dependent individuals. Some compounds also appear to block drug cue–induced craving that relates to relapse. These medications include DA releasers such as sustained-release formulations of medications used to treat attention-deficit/hyperactivity disorder; mixed DA reuptake inhibitors (modafinil); DA precursors (L-dopa); NE synthesis blockers (disulfiram); and drugs that potentiate GLU neurotransmission (N-acetylcysteine). The difficulty of defining the appropriate therapeutic target to produce positive clinical results, as well as the cost of development, has led to inadequate involvement by the pharmaceutical industry. Although some agonist therapies have shown promising results, it remains controversial whether their potential abuse liability would outweigh their possible clinical efficacy.

Chapter 6 covers polydrug abuse. Substance abuse comorbidity is common with alcohol, marijuana, and opiates. Common psychiatric comorbidity includes depression, psychosis, and personality disorders.

Medical comorbidity and HIV are addressed in Chapter 7. A substantial problem with medical comorbidity is that despite evident extreme examples of health problems resulting from cocaine or METH use, these comorbid conditions often are not credible to users. Many well-controlled studies link stimulant use to a number of medical problems, some of which are fatal. Knowledge of these problems can help stimulant users and health care providers respond to symptoms earlier, but the denial of these major medical complications among the stimulant users is a significant challenge.

The list of complications begins with stimulant overdose (Centers for Disease Control and Prevention 2010), which manifests initially with symptoms such as agitation, increased heart rate, and hyperthermia (Kosten and Kleber 1988). Hyperthermia is particularly lethal through progression to rhabdomyolysis and renal failure. Long-term stimulant use increases the risk of hypertension, atherosclerosis, vasospasm, thrombosis formation, myocardial infarction, and stroke. Rarely, vasoconstriction can also cause corneal ulcers and scarring, resulting in blindness. Smoking crack or METH harms the lungs, exacerbates asthma and chronic obstructive pulmonary disease, and increases vulnerability to tuberculosis. Cocaine and especially METH can cause gum disease and tooth decay via vasoconstriction, dehydration, reduced salivary flow, poor dental hygiene, and poor diet. Cocaine and METH use can lead to dehydration and nutritional deficiencies that result in dry, itchy skin. In addition, some users have tactile or visual hallucinations involving their skin (e.g., feeling bugs under their skin) that exacerbates damage to the skin through their picking at it (Gawin and Ellinwood 1988).

Behavioral complications of chronic stimulants extend from the neonatal and pediatric periods to older adulthood (Delaney-Black et al. 2010). Children who are exposed prenatally to cocaine or METH are at increased risk for neurobehavioral problems and should receive regular developmental and mental health assessments and referrals as needed. Cocaine and METH use is associated with increased risk of violence toward and from intimate partners, even after other risk factors are taken into account. Unprotected sex and the reuse of previously used needles, syringes, and possibly pipes can transmit HIV and hepatitis C virus. Poor skin hygiene when injecting can result in infections of the skin (abscesses), heart (endocarditis), or other organs. The adulterant levamisole, found in most cocaine, can result in neutropenia and life-threatening infections. Finally, cocaine and possibly METH increase HIV disease progression, even after taking into account other risk factors. To reduce this disparity, it is important to engage stimulant users in HIV care and addiction treatment as early as possible.

The continued high levels of cocaine and METH/AMPH abuse and the destructive effects of such abuse call for renewed efforts to improve treatment results. This comprehensive volume brings together what is known about these drugs and points the way to such improvement. As such, it is an important contribution to the addiction field.

Herbert D. Kleber, M.D.
Professor of Psychiatry and Director, Division of Substance Abuse,
Columbia University, New York, New York

References

Aharonovich E, Nunes E, Hasin D: Cognitive impairment, retention and abstinence among cocaine abusers in cognitive-behavioral treatment. Drug Alcohol Depend 71:207–211, 2003

Aharonovich E, Hasin DS, Brooks AC, et al: Cognitive deficits predict low treatment retention in cocaine dependent patients. Drug Alcohol Depend 81:313–322, 2006

Ahmad K: Asia grapples with spreading amphetamine abuse. Lancet 361:1878–1879, 2003

Carroll KM: Integrating psychotherapy and pharmacotherapy to improve drug abuse outcomes. Addict Behav 22:233–245, 1997

Carroll KM, Nich C, Ball SA, et al: One-year follow-up of disulfiram and psychotherapy for cocaine-alcohol users: sustained effects of treatment. Addiction 95:1335–1349, 2000

Centers for Disease Control and Prevention: Unintentional drug poisoning in the United States. July 2010. Available at: http://www.cdc.gov/HomeandRecreationalSafety/pdf/poison-issue-brief.pdf. Accessed March 15, 2011.

Crits-Christoph P, Siqueland L, Blaine J, et al: Psychosocial treatments for cocaine dependence: National Institute on Drug Abuse Collaborative Cocaine Treatment Study. Arch Gen Psychiatry 56:493–502, 1999

Delaney-Black V, Chiodo LM, Hannigan JH, et al: Just say "I don't": lack of concordance between teen report and biological measures of drug use. Pediatrics 126:887–893, 2010

Galanter M, Kleber HD (eds): The American Psychiatric Publishing Textbook of Substance Abuse Treatment, 4th Edition. Washington, DC, American Psychiatric Publishing, 2008

Gawin FH, Ellinwood EHJ: Cocaine and other stimulants: actions, abuse, and treatment. N Engl J Med 318:1173–1182, 1988

Gay GR: Clinical management of acute and chronic cocaine poisoning. Ann Emerg Med 11:562–572, 1982

Graham JK, Hanzlick R: Accidental drug deaths in Fulton County, Georgia, 2002: characteristics, case management and certification issues. Am J Forensic Med Pathol 29:224–230, 2008

Grassi MC, Cioce AM, Giudici FD, et al: Short-term efficacy of disulfiram or naltrexone in reducing positive urinalysis for both cocaine and cocaethylene in cocaine abusers: a pilot study. Pharmacol Res 55:117–121, 2007

Higgins ST, Budney AJ, Bickel WK, et al: Incentives improve outcome in outpatient behavioral treatment of cocaine dependence. Arch Gen Psychiatry 51:568–576, 1994a

Higgins ST, Budney AJ, Bickel WK, et al: Participation of significant others in outpatient behavioral treatment predicts greater cocaine abstinence. Am J Drug Alcohol Abuse 20:47–56, 1994b

Higgins ST, Badger GJ, Budney AJ: Initial abstinence and success in achieving longer term cocaine abstinence. Exp Clin Psychopharmacol 8:377–386, 2000a

Higgins ST, Wong CJ, Badger GJ, et al: Contingent reinforcement increases cocaine abstinence during outpatient treatment and 1 year of follow-up. J Consult Clin Psychol 68:64–72, 2000b

Hughes JR, Hatsukami DK, Mitchell JE, et al: Prevalence of smoking among psychiatric outpatients. Am J Psychiatry 143:993–997, 1986

Jacobsen LK, Southwick SM, Kosten TR: Substance use disorders in patients with posttraumatic stress disorder: a review of the literature. Am J Psychiatry 158:1184–1190, 2001

Johnston L, O'Malley P, Bachman J, et al: Monitoring the Future: national survey results on drug use, 1975–2009, Vol I: Secondary School Students (NIH Publ No 10-7584). Bethesda, MD, National Institute on Drug Abuse, 2010

Kaye S, Darke S, Duflou J, et al: Methamphetamine-related fatalities in Australia: demographics, circumstances, toxicology and major organ pathology. Addiction 103:1353–1360, 2008

Kosten TR, Kleber HD: Rapid death during cocaine abuse: a variant of the neuroleptic malignant syndrome? Am J Drug Alcohol Abuse 14:335–346, 1988

McLellan AT, Lewis DC, O'Brien CP, et al: Drug dependence, a chronic medical illness: implications for treatment, insurance, and outcomes evaluation. JAMA 284:1689–1695, 2000

Olmstead TA, Ostrow CD, Carroll KM: Cost-effectiveness of computer-assisted training in cognitive-behavioral therapy as an adjunct to standard care for addiction. Drug Alcohol Depend 110:200–207, 2010

Petry NM: Methadone plus contingency management or performance feedback reduces cocaine and opiate use in people with drug addiction. Evid Based Ment Health 8:112, 2005

Poling J, Oliveto A, Petry N, et al: Six-month trial of bupropion with contingency management for cocaine dependence in a methadone-maintained population. Arch Gen Psychiatry 63:219–228, 2006

Rawson RA, McCann MJ, Flammino F, et al: A comparison of contingency management and cognitive-behavioral approaches for stimulant-dependent individuals. Addiction 101:267–274, 2006

Silverman K, Higgins ST, Brooner RK, et al: Sustained cocaine abstinence in methadone maintenance patients through voucher-based reinforcement therapy. Arch Gen Psychiatry 53:409–415, 1996

Substance Abuse and Mental Health Services Administration: Drug Abuse Warning Network, 2007: national estimates of drug-related emergency department visits. 2010a. Available at: http://dawninfo.samhsa.gov/files/ed2007/dawn2k7ed.pdf. Accessed March 15, 2011.

Substance Abuse and Mental Health Services Administration: Results from the 2009 National Survey on Drug Use and Health, Vol I: Summary of National Findings (Office of Applied Studies, NSDUH Series H-38A, HHS Publ No SMA 10-4586). 2010b. Available at: http://www.oas.samhsa.gov/NSDUH/2k9NSDUH/2k9ResultsP.pdf. Accessed March 15, 2011.

Substance Abuse and Mental Health Services Administration: Treatment Episode Data Set (TEDS): 1998–2008. National Admissions to Substance Abuse Treatment Services (Office of Applied Studies, DASIS Series S-50, HHS Publ No SMA-09-4471). 2010c. Available at: http://wwwdasis.samhsa.gov/teds08/teds2k8natweb.pdf. Accessed March 15, 2011.

Volkow ND, Fowler JS, Wolf AP, et al: Effects of chronic cocaine abuse on postsynaptic dopamine receptors. Am J Psychiatry 147:719–724, 1990

Weinstock J, Alessi SM, Petry NM: Regardless of psychiatric severity the addition of contingency management to standard treatment improves retention and drug use outcomes. Drug Alcohol Depend 87:288–296, 2007

Chapter 1

Epidemiology and Psychiatric Comorbidity

Thomas R. Kosten, M.D.
Thomas F. Newton, M.D.

Epidemiology and Background

The epidemiology of cocaine, amphetamine (AMPH), and methamphetamine (METH) abuse and dependence reflects substantial differences in distribution, with cocaine being supplied through ports of entry from sources in South America and AMPH and METH coming from more "home-grown" sources, at least until recently. Cocaine from Colombia and its neighboring countries typically arrived in urban areas, where its use became epidemic in North American cities in the 1980s. Cocaine was rarely exported to rural areas. Now, increasing amounts of cocaine are being smuggled through the Mexican border into California, Arizona, and Texas, although cocaine, unlike METH, remains primarily an urban problem. Most METH is now imported into the United States from Mexico, and METH from this source is fast replacing METH of local manufacture, which predominated until the later 2000s. This shift in distribution appears to be due to policies initiated to restrict importation of precursor chemicals such as pseudoephedrine into the United States, whereas such chemicals continue to be imported into Mexico.

1

A steady decline in U.S. METH lab seizures from 2004 to 2007 with a slight increase in 2008 reflects aggressive policing measures.

METH distribution networks are separate from those for cocaine, with METH predominating in rural, western, and southern regions of the United States. Information on geographic trends in drug abuse comes from sources such as the National Institute on Drug Abuse Community Epidemiology Work Group, which in June 2009 reported that primary METH abuse treatment admissions were declining for nearly all U.S. cities being monitored (Figure 1–1) (National Institute on Drug Abuse 2010). This decline likely stems from reductions in local production, as noted above.

This geographic distribution for abuse of these drugs can also be shown through community-wide drug testing of wastewater samples as a population measure of community drug use. Such studies indicate that cocaine use peaks at weekends, as would be expected given its generally intermittent use. A report of a Belgian study of cocaine index wastewater loads (milligrams/ person/day) included a map suggesting greater urban than rural use, as was also found in an Oregon study of cocaine metabolites, which were significantly higher in urban areas and below detection in many rural areas (Banta-Green et al. 2009). Conversely, METH was present in the wastewater of all Oregon municipalities, with no significant differences in index loads by urban versus rural area. Wastewater METH index loads also indicate higher usage of METH in the United States than in Europe, which is consistent with findings from other epidemiological surveys. Overall, the fast-moving and geographically influenced trends in abuse epidemics of METH and cocaine are difficult to monitor in real time with existing drug use indicators, and these novel public health approaches are finding some use for projections of drug-related crime levels and prevention and treatment needs.

Our chapter is focused on the current cocaine epidemic and its course, but this is not the first epidemic of cocaine use in the United States, as documented by David Musto in his classic book *The American Disease.* Cocaine was a significant public health problem as early as the turn of the twentieth century and led to drastically punitive legal measures (Musto 1999). The more recent U.S. epidemic, spanning the 1980s, also produced a substantial criminal justice response but has resulted in more humane linkages between the criminal justice system and treatment. Examples include "drug courts," where judges offer the convicted cocaine or METH abuser the option of engaging in legally supervised treatment rather than going to prison. Treatment has also been introduced into the prisons themselves and includes options for reducing the duration of imprisonment through work-release programs. These work-release programs allow legally supervised treatment beyond the typical limitations of parole programs, with their overwhelming caseloads of 400 or more parolees per supervisor.

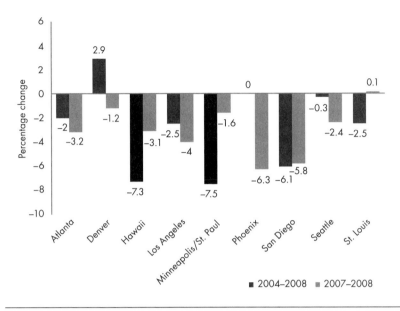

FIGURE 1–1. Primary methamphetamine treatment admissions in nine Community Epidemiology Work Group reporting areas as a percentage of primary drug admissions, excluding primary alcohol admissions.
Source. National Institute on Drug Abuse 2010.

Other legal interventions have been less enlightened. Most notable is the establishment of substantially more severe penalties for crack than for powder cocaine possession and sale. Crack cocaine is the base form of the drug, whereas powder cocaine is the hydrochloride salt. These two forms of cocaine are pharmacologically equivalent and have the same addictive potential. Such a distinction in penalties seems to reflect a bias against minorities, as inner-city cocaine abusers are more likely than suburban whites to smoke and sell the crack form of the drug. Thus, we have made some sociopolitical progress in our approach to the abuse and the abusers of stimulants, but more enlightened policies and approaches to demand reduction beyond policing are needed.

The U.S. cocaine epidemic had its peak in 1985 and produced an estimated 2.5 million lifetime stimulant abusers. We now have about 1.4 million current cocaine abusers and 350,000 current AMPH abusers (Johnston et al. 2010a). These 2.5 million lifetime abusers contribute some long-term users to the total, from the peak of the epidemic 25 years ago, but a steady stream of new users also adds to the current number of users. Between 1991 and 1998, the 30-day prevalence of cocaine abuse among eighth, tenth, and twelfth graders increased more than twofold, and the 2009 Monitoring the Future study of

U.S. secondary students found that 3.4% of twelfth graders had used cocaine in the previous year and 1.3% had used crack (Johnston et al. 2010b).

Casualties from stimulant use also continue to accumulate, as cocaine involvement in emergency department (ED) accident and violence cases remains prominent. Drug Abuse Warning Network (DAWN) 2009 data, derived from representative EDs, shows 482,000 mentions of cocaine compared with 1,000,000 for alcohol and 1,900,000 for all legal and illegal drugs (Substance Abuse and Mental Health Services Administration 2010). The number of deaths from cocaine overdose has also risen steadily, from 3,500 in 1999 to 7,000 in 2006 (Centers for Disease Control and Prevention 2010). The numbers of new abusers of cocaine, stimulants (including METH), and ecstasy (3,4-methylenedioxymethamphetamine; MDMA) remain high compared with the number of new users of marijuana, as shown in Table 1–1. Overall, cocaine dependence complications are common, involving one of every three drug-related ED visits, and cocaine has substantial social and economic impacts on those afflicted (McLellan et al. 2000; Substance Abuse and Mental Health Services Administration 2010). From 2007 through 2009, the United States had 2.5 million cocaine abusers, and only 809,000 of them were treated in 2007 (Johnston et al. 2010a).

This endemic cocaine abuse in North and South America has more recently spread to Europe, starting in Spain as an epidemic in about the year 2000. This introduction into Spain is not surprising, given the commonality in language with South America. Cocaine abuse has spread rapidly to the rest of Europe and Great Britain, particularly among comorbid opiate abusers who have been injecting amphetamines for many years.

METH abuse is an international public health problem, with two-thirds of the world's 33 million AMPH abusers living in Asia (Ahmad 2003). In Hong Kong, the prevalence of AMPH abuse rose from 1% in 1995 to 17% in 2000. The largest producers of METH are in Southeast Asia and North America, where the majority of users reside (Ahmad 2003). Localized epidemics of METH abuse have developed, particularly in the western United States. The Philippines have the world's highest rates of METH abuse, with an estimated 2.9% or more of the population being abusers. Because of this high rate, METH is the primary drug of concern in the Philippines and several nearby countries in Southeast Asia. A growing market is emerging in South Africa.

AMPH (as opposed to METH) production and use occur primarily in Europe, where injection use is common. Prevalence rates range from 0.7% of the population in Western Europe to 0.2% in Eastern and southern Europe. In the United States, AMPH was available over the counter in inhalers until 1959. AMPH abuse from diverted pharmaceutical sources was a significant problem until 1970, when the drug was moved to the more restrictive Drug Enforcement Agency Schedule II.

TABLE 1–1. Past-year initiates for cocaine, ecstasy, stimulants, and marijuana among persons age 12 or older in 2007

Drug	New abusers
Cocaine	906,000
Ecstasy	781,000
Stimulants	642,000
Marijuana	2,090,000

Source. Substance Abuse and Mental Health Services Administration, Office of Applied Studies, National Survey on Drug Use and Health, 2008.

Abuse of METH has been consistently much more prevalent in the United States since the 1990s, when large quantities of a highly pure, smoked form of METH began to be imported from Asia to Hawaii and then to the West Coast of the United States.

The history and epidemiology of METH in the United States starts with these imported supplies from Asia and then moves to METH production on Mexico and California. A rapid increase in small clandestine laboratories on the West Coast and in the Midwest reached its peak in 2003–2004, when more than 16,000 laboratory incidents per year were recorded. This rate fell dramatically to about 5,000 per year by 2007 as law enforcement efforts to control supplies of the ephedrine precursors and to find and destroy these laboratories were effective (Johnston et al. 2010b). These efforts increased the price of METH by over 80%, while its purity decreased by 26%, and the indicators in almost all metropolitan areas showed stable or reduced use of METH. The national Monitoring the Future study in 2007 also showed a substantial reduction in METH use by twelfth graders, from 2.6% in 2006 to 1.6% in 2007 (Johnston et al. 2010b). Moreover, more recent data from this study in 2009 showed a continued decline in METH use, to 1.2% (Johnston et al. 2010a).

In contrast to this remarkable and rapid reduction in METH use related to these legal interventions, medical and psychiatric complications of METH abuse increased over the longer period from 1995 to 2007. Much of this increase was associated with METH production in Mexico. States on both sides of the Mexican–U.S. border have had substantial increases in METH treatment admissions during these 12 years, from 7% to 25% in Mexico and from 12% to 27% in the U.S. border states. This increased rate of METH admissions was most prominent for western Mexico, while eastern Mexico and Texas had a predominant increase in cocaine treatment admissions during this period.

The abuser often notices few negative health consequences from METH or other stimulants, such as cocaine, but epidemiological data show that serious medical problems are relatively common and can occur suddenly or insidiously. Coroners' reports (Graham and Hanzlick 2008; Kaye et al. 2008) relate stimulants to the direct cause of death in 25% of cocaine overdoses and 68% of METH overdoses or identify stimulants as antecedents to cardiovascular or other medical problems, leading to death in 20% of abusers who overdose. In later chapters, the authors review the most common medical consequences of cocaine and METH use, including overdose, cumulative effects on various organ systems, behavior changes resulting in injuries, and infectious diseases such as AIDS and hepatitis.

A significant change in the main route of administration for METH occurred from the early epidemic in 1995 to 2007; abusers shifted from inhaled (50% to 15%) to smoked (12% to 66%) METH. This shift to a more rapid route of administration increased METH reinforcement, the amount used, and the associated toxicity during binges of abuse. The consequence of this shift in route of administration included treatment admissions going up nearly 10-fold from 1995 to 2007, representing 9% of all national drug-related treatment admissions. The demographics also shifted between 1995 and 2007, to include more minorities needing treatment, as the percentage of patients admitted for METH treatment who were white changed from over 90% to 70% and the percentage of patients who were Hispanic doubled, from 9% to 19%. Admissions for METH continued to be about half males and half females during this 12-year period. The greatest rates of admission for METH in the United States in 2007 were in Hawaii (244/100,000 population) and California (218/100,000). Deaths were also concentrated in these western states, as reported by DAWN (Substance Abuse and Mental Health Services Administration 2010).

Populations at high risk for METH abuse include Native Americans, the homeless, the gay community, and sex workers. Among Native Americans, only inhalants and alcohol surpass METH in terms of treatment admissions, and primary care encounters at Indian Health Service facilities related to METH abuse increased 250% from 2000 to 2005. The homeless are also at high risk for METH abuse, with a recent study in Los Angeles finding that a quarter of the city's homeless population had used METH (National Institute on Drug Abuse 2010). Among the white homeless persons, 60% had used METH. The abuse of METH in gay communities is strongly associated with sexual risk behaviors for contracting HIV infections. The rate of METH or other stimulant use from 2000 to 2005 doubled, to 22% among HIV-infected gay men in the southern United States. High-risk sexual behaviors include unprotected receptive anal sex. Female sex workers are also more likely to use METH than to use other drugs, and heterosexual METH abusers are more likely than heterosexual non-METH abusers to engage in a wide range of HIV risk behaviors. METH use in the workplace more generally, including among long-distance truck drivers, remains a concern, but there are insufficient data. However, paralleling the apparent success of the legal interventions in 2007 in reducing METH supplies, the incidence of workplace urine samples testing positive for METH, which had been steadily rising through 2006, declined by 50% in 2007.

As noted earlier, in our discussion of the 2009 Monitoring the Future study results, METH abuse had declined to 1.6% and cocaine abuse was relatively stable at 3.4%, but the study also showed that 6.6% of twelfth graders had used AMPH in the previous year (Johnston et al. 2010b). This suggests a trend toward increasing nonmedical use of AMPH from pharmaceutical sources, substituting for METH made in local U.S. clandestine laboratories or imported from Mexico. In fact, prescriptions of stimulants dispensed by U.S. retail pharmacies from 1999 to 2009 rose from 4 million to 39 million, representing an almost 10-fold increase in supplies available for diversion to abuse.

Overall, the changing epidemiology of stimulant abuse, resulting from an increase in pharmaceutical abuse, is due to several factors:

1. An increasing number of prescriptions has led to greater availability.
2. Attention by the media to this form of abuse and advertising on television and in newspapers have stimulated adolescents' interest in this abuse.
3. Easy access to stimulants through family and friends has made this type of abuse cheap and attractive.
4. Insufficient knowledge and monitoring of adolescents and of disappearance of drugs in the home or elsewhere has meant that addiction has gone unrecognized.

In spite of these unrecognized addictions, the dangers associated with stimulant use are enormous and include increased risk of HIV infection, possible detrimental effects on the fetus and newborn, increased crime and violence, and medical, financial, and psychological problems.

Comorbidity With Psychiatric Diseases

Cocaine and METH abuse and dependence frequently co-occur with other major (i.e., Axis I) mental illnesses, especially schizophrenia, major depression (Hughes et al. 1986), and posttraumatic stress disorder (PTSD) (Jacobsen et al. 2001). Although cocaine and METH are both stimulants, they differ significantly in their clinical effects (Mahoney et al. 2008; Newton et al.

2005). They also differ in which populations they affect most (Banta-Green et al. 2009). For these reasons, it is most useful to consider these drugs separately. Our main focus here will be on mental illnesses occurring in populations selected for cocaine and METH use, although we will briefly cover drug use occurring in populations selected for mental illness.

In a study of 303 crack cocaine users, most of whom (59.7%) met criteria for cocaine dependence, Falck and colleagues reported that 17.8% met criteria for major depression and 11.8% met criteria for PTSD (Falck et al. 2004). These rates are more than double those reported in the general population (Kessler et al. 2005). Unlike in the general population, rates of depression did not differ between male and female cocaine users. Females did have a higher prevalence of PTSD (18.9% vs. 7.0%), possibly reflecting higher levels of trauma among women. Attention-deficit/hyperactivity disorder was also present at relatively high rates (9.9%), as were phobias (9.9%) and panic disorder (3.8%). Other disorders, such as schizophrenia and generalized anxiety disorder, were present at low rates. This study used the Diagnostic Interview Schedule to make DSM-IV diagnoses, and this approach generally yields valid estimates of prevalence.

Cocaine dependence frequently co-occurs with other drug use disorders. In a large study, nearly half of cocaine-dependent participants also had lifetime diagnoses of alcohol dependence (49.7%) or opioid dependence (45.3%), and fewer had lifetime diagnoses of cannabis dependence (30.1%). Less than 10% had lifetime diagnoses of sedative or other stimulant use (Ford et al. 2009). Most cocaine users also smoke cigarettes (Roll et al. 1996).

This same study (Ford et al. 2009) found that many METH users also meet the criteria for alcohol dependence. About 18.8% of those with comorbid psychosis met the alcohol dependence criteria, whereas only 6.1% of those without comorbid psychosis met the criteria. There is less information available about cannabis use, though our impression is that it is relatively more common among METH users compared with cocaine users. Like cocaine users, most METH users smoke cigarettes (De La Garza et al. 2008).

METH users appear to be at a higher risk for developing psychotic symptoms. In a study of 431 METH users in Taiwan, Chen and colleagues (2003) reported that 39% had experienced psychotic symptoms in the past. Among the subgroup recruited from psychiatric hospitals, nearly 26.4% had prolonged psychotic symptoms after stopping METH use, whereas the remaining subjects (who were recruited from police custody) had very low rates of psychotic symptoms. Most reports of high rates of psychosis among METH users are from Asia, though it is unknown whether this distribution represents a real difference in susceptibility or an ascertainment bias, with Asians simply reporting on psychosis more frequently.

Other disorders are more prevalent among METH users. Pathological gambling was present in 12.4% of those with comorbid psychosis ($n=261$) and only 4.2% of those without comorbid psychosis ($n=170$) (Chen et al. 2003). Depression was present in 7.6% of those with comorbid psychosis and 3.8% of those without comorbid psychosis. This study used the Diagnostic Interview for Genetic Studies, which is generally considered valid and reliable to diagnose comorbid psychiatric disorders.

Cocaine withdrawal was discussed at length in the 1980s, and substantial clinical importance was attached to it (Gawin and Kleber 1986). Since then, however, it has been shown that cocaine withdrawal symptoms are minimal during monitored abstinence (Weddington et al. 1990). A modified conceptualization of cocaine withdrawal has been described that emphasizes changes in appetite, sleep, and mood (Kampman et al. 1998), and scores on this scale appear to correlate with outcome and treatment response (Kampman et al. 2002). Thus, while cocaine withdrawal may be associated with only modest symptoms, there is preliminary evidence that these may have clinical significance.

Contrary to a common lay misconception, cessation of METH use generally produces a relatively mild withdrawal syndrome that resolves over a week or so (McGregor et al. 2005; Newton et al. 2004). Some people do develop more severe symptoms, and this response can be associated with the development of major depression in a minority of users (Glasner-Edwards et al. 2008). Symptoms are most prominent in the first several days of abstinence, and this may prompt users to relapse to ongoing METH use at an early point during a quit attempt.

Drug use is more common among patients with mental illnesses than among the general population. For example, Shaner and colleagues (1993) found over 30% of patients with schizophrenia tested positive for cocaine on admission to the hospital. Nicotine use is nearly ubiquitous among severely mentally ill individuals. In a classic study, Hughes and colleagues reported that 88% of outpatients with schizophrenia smoked cigarettes, and patients with bipolar disorder had similar rates (Hughes et al. 1986). Patients with mood and anxiety disorders were at less risk for smoking but still smoked at higher rates than did control subjects. Although further discussion of such findings is beyond the scope of this chapter, the explanation for these associations is undoubtedly complex, involving a host of biological and social factors.

KEY CLINICAL CONCEPTS

- Laws enacted in the United States to regulate precursor chemicals used to manufacture methamphetamine (METH) and amphetamine (AMPH), with aggressive policing, resulted in decreased drug availability, but it appears that production of these drugs has shifted to Mexico, and supplies remain high.

- Production of METH has shifted somewhat to the Midwest, where small-scale laboratories provide limited product, but Mexican laboratories are still the source of most METH.

- Most of the world's METH/AMPH abusers reside in Southeast Asia and North America, with the Philippines having the highest rates.

- The cocaine epidemic in the United States peaked in 1985. There were an estimated 1.4 million current cocaine users during 2008. Deaths due to cocaine overdose have continued to increase.

- METH/AMPH abuse is declining in high school–aged users, yet there is increasing use of diverted prescription stimulants.

- More humane policies by the criminal justice system, moving away from punitive action and toward medical management and treatment for drug dependence–related infractions, represent a major step that may decrease numbers of long-term drug abusers.

- Major mental illness, such as depression and psychosis, is common in METH/AMPH-dependent individuals. Psychotic symptoms often do not abate after the individual stops using the drug, and the individual tends to be dependent on other substances, such as alcohol and nicotine.

- Major depression, posttraumatic stress disorder, attention-deficit/hyperactivity disorder, phobias, and panic disorder are more prevalent in cocaine-dependent individuals, and these individuals are usually dependent on other drugs, such as alcohol, opioids, and nicotine.

- Contrary to what is generally assumed, withdrawal from cocaine and METH/AMPH is relatively mild and short in duration, but a small proportion of users do develop major depression in withdrawal.

- Drug use is much more common in individuals with mental illness compared with the general population.

Resources

http://www.nida.nih.gov/about/organization/cewg/Reports.html
http://ondcp.gov/publications/asp/topics.asp
http://monitoringthefuture.org/

References

Ahmad K: Asia grapples with spreading amphetamine abuse. Lancet 361:1878–1879, 2003

Banta-Green CJ, Field JA, Chiaia AC, et al: The spatial epidemiology of cocaine, methamphetamine and 3,4-methylenedioxymethamphetamine (MDMA) use: a demonstration using a population measure of community drug load derived from municipal wastewater. Addiction 104:1874–1880, 2009

Centers for Disease Control and Prevention: Unintentional drug poisoning in the United States. July 2010. Available at: http://www.cdc.gov/HomeandRecreationalSafety/pdf/poison-issue-brief.pdf. Accessed March 15, 2011.

Chen CK, Lin SK, Sham PC, et al: Pre-morbid characteristics and co-morbidity of methamphetamine users with and without psychosis. Psychol Med 33:1407–1414, 2003

De La Garza R 2nd, Mahoney JJ 3rd, Culbertson C, et al: The acetylcholinesterase inhibitor rivastigmine does not alter total choices for methamphetamine, but may reduce positive subjective effects, in a laboratory model of intravenous self-administration in human volunteers. Pharmacol Biochem Behav 89:200–208, 2008

Falck RS, Wang J, Siegal HA, et al: The prevalence of psychiatric disorder among a community sample of crack cocaine users: an exploratory study with practical implications. J Nerv Ment Dis 192:503–507, 2004

Ford JD, Gelernter J, DeVoe JS, et al: Association of psychiatric and substance use disorder comorbidity with cocaine dependence severity and treatment utilization in cocaine-dependent individuals. Drug Alcohol Depend 99:193–203, 2009

Gawin FH, Kleber HD: Abstinence symptomatology and psychiatric diagnosis in cocaine abusers. Clinical observations. Arch Gen Psychiatry 43:107–113, 1986

Glasner-Edwards S, Mooney LJ, Marinelli-Casey P, et al: Identifying methamphetamine users at risk for major depressive disorder: findings from the Methamphetamine Treatment Project at three-year follow-up. Am J Addict 17:99–102, 2008

Graham JK, Hanzlick R: Accidental drug deaths in Fulton County, Georgia, 2002: characteristics, case management and certification issues. Am J Forensic Med Pathol 29:224–230, 2008

Hughes JR, Hatsukami DK, Mitchell JE, et al: Prevalence of smoking among psychiatric outpatients. Am J Psychiatry 143:993–997, 1986

Jacobsen LK, Southwick SM, Kosten TR: Substance use disorders in patients with posttraumatic stress disorder: a review of the literature. Am J Psychiatry 158:1184–1190, 2001

Johnston L, O'Malley P, Bachman J, et al: Monitoring the Future: National Survey Results on Adolescent Drug Use: Overview of Key Findings, 2009 (NIH Publ No 10-7583). Bethesda, MD, National Institute on Drug Abuse, 2010a

Johnston L, O'Malley P, Bachman J, et al: Monitoring the Future: National Survey Results on Drug Use, 1975–2009, Vol I: Secondary School Students (NIH Publ No 10-7584). Bethesda, MD, National Institute on Drug Abuse, 2010b

Kampman KM, Volpicelli JR, McGinnis DE, et al: Reliability and validity of the Cocaine Selective Severity Assessment. Addict Behav 23:449–461, 1998

Kampman KM, Volpicelli JR, Mulvaney F, et al: Cocaine withdrawal severity and urine toxicology results from treatment entry predict outcome in medication trials for cocaine dependence. Addict Behav 27:251–260, 2002

Kaye S, Darke S, Duflou J, et al: Methamphetamine-related fatalities in Australia: demographics, circumstances, toxicology and major organ pathology. Addiction 103:1353–1360, 2008

Kessler RC, Chiu WT, Demler O, et al: Prevalence, severity, and comorbidity of 12-month DSM-IV disorders in the National Comorbidity Survey Replication. Arch Gen Psychiatry 62:617–627, 2005

Mahoney JJ 3rd, Kalechstein AD, De La Garza R 2nd, et al: Presence and persistence of psychotic symptoms in cocaine- versus methamphetamine-dependent participants. Am J Addict 17:83–98, 2008

McGregor C, Srisurapanont M, Jittiwutikarn J, et al: The nature, time course and severity of methamphetamine withdrawal. Addiction 100:1320–1329, 2005

McLellan AT, Lewis DC, O'Brien CP, et al: Drug dependence, a chronic medical illness: implications for treatment, insurance, and outcomes evaluation. JAMA 284:1689–1695, 2000

Musto DF: The American Disease: Origins of Narcotic Control, 3rd Edition. New York, Oxford University Press, 1999

National Institute on Drug Abuse, Community Epidemiology Work Group (CEWG): Epidemiologic Trends in Drug Abuse: Proceedings of the Community Epidemiology Work Group, Volume 1: Highlights and Executive Summary, June 2009 (NIH Publ No 10-7421). Bethesda, MD, U.S. Department of Health and Human Services, National Institutes of Health, 2010

Newton TF, Kalechstein AD, Duran S, et al: Methamphetamine abstinence syndrome: preliminary findings. Am J Addict 13:248–255, 2004

Newton TF, De La Garza R 2nd, Kalechstein AD, et al: Cocaine and methamphetamine produce different patterns of subjective and cardiovascular effects. Pharmacol Biochem Behav 82:90–97, 2005

Roll JM, Higgins ST, Budney AJ, et al: A comparison of cocaine-dependent cigarette smokers and non-smokers on demographic, drug use and other characteristics. Drug Alcohol Depend 40:195–201, 1996

Shaner A, Khalsa ME, Roberts L, et al: Unrecognized cocaine use among schizophrenic patients. Am J Psychiatry 150:758–762, 1993

Substance Abuse and Mental Health Services Administration: Drug Abuse Warning Network, 2007: national estimates of drug-related emergency department visits. 2010. Available at: http://dawninfo.samhsa.gov/files/ed2007/dawn2k7ed.pdf. Accessed March 15, 2011.

Weddington WW, Brown BS, Haertzen CA, et al: Changes in mood, craving, and sleep during short-term abstinence reported by male cocaine addicts. A controlled, residential study. Arch Gen Psychiatry 47:861–868, 1990

Chapter 2

History, Use, and Basic Pharmacology of Stimulants

Colin N. Haile, M.D., Ph.D.

Humans have been altering their consciousness with botanical and chemical substances for thousands of years (El-Seedi et al. 2005). Stimulants in particular have long been used for their energizing properties and many have indications for medical use today. Nontherapeutic use of stimulants and consequences secondary to abuse continue to be a pernicious problem. Indeed, a recent United States National Survey on Drug Use and Health noted that stimulant addiction accounted for 17% of all patients who entered treatment programs (Substance Abuse and Mental Health Services Administration 2010). With the exception of some behavioral strategies, there are presently no efficacious treatments for stimulant dependence (Rawson et al. 2004; Vocci and Montoya 2009). Much progress in our understanding has been achieved through basic biochemical research and with animal models of different characteristics of human drug dependence. Even more insight has been gained through advances in neuroimaging technology that have been pivotal in furthering our understanding of areas of the brain in which stimulants exert their potent reinforcing effects.

This chapter presents a general overview of the basic pharmacological and neurochemical actions of cocaine, methamphetamine (METH), and amphetamine (AMPH). Anatomical structures, brain circuitry, neurotransmitter systems, and molecular mechanisms central to their effects are reviewed. Drug pharmacokinetics and pharmacodynamics are surveyed in relation to stimulant dependence and the development of possible pharmacotherapies. A brief history of each drug is also included to foster appreciation of their legal and illicit use over time. This examination is by no means exhaustive, and the reader is pointed to more comprehensive and original publications for detailed information. It is hoped that this chapter does, however, provide the reader with a greater understanding of how these highly addictive drugs affect the brain and what advances have been made in the development of possible treatments for psychostimulant dependence.

Important Definitions in Drug Dependence and Behavioral Pharmacology

Hallmark characteristics of substance dependence and abuse are detailed elsewhere in this book. I discuss here a few that directly apply to this chapter—namely, drug seeking and drug intake known to be detrimental and not in the individual's best interest that is continued despite deteriorating physical, mental health and social footing (see Table 2–1). *Drug dependence* broadly describes substance-seeking behavior, inability to stop using, and incremental increases in drug intake. The need to increase drug intake over time indicates *tolerance,* which is usually ascribed to the drug's pleasurable and peripheral physiological effects. Physiological and/or psychological dependence are also characteristics of drug dependence. *Physiological dependence* results when a withdrawal syndrome involving physiological and/or psychological components occurs when drug intake ceases. Other important pharmacological concepts include *cross-tolerance,* or tolerance to one substance that develops also to another substance in the same class. Under certain circumstances, stimulants such as cocaine and METH can induce *sensitization.* That is, a drug dose can produce greater behavioral effects upon multiple exposures over time. Like cross-tolerance, cross-sensitization can occur between drugs in the same class.

TABLE 2–1. Important definitions

Substance abuse	Use of a substance has led to impairment or distress that may include failure to meet work, school, or home obligations; use during hazardous activities; recurrent substance-related legal issues; and continued use despite obvious problems.
Substance dependence	
Tolerance	A decreased response to a drug that requires increased doses to achieve initial effects. Metabolic, behavioral and functional tolerance may play a role.
Withdrawal	Substance-specific syndrome after cessation or reduction in the amount of substance used that is clinically significant and causes distress or impairment.

Neuropharmacology

Neurobiological Substrates, Neurotransmission, and Molecular Machinery

The motivating or reinforcing (i.e., euphoric) effects produced by stimulants are mediated by many brain areas and neurotransmitter systems. Studies strongly support activation of the mesocorticolimbic dopamine (DA) system as key to governing stimulants' reinforcing effects. Yet other neurotransmitter systems, including norepinephrine (NE), epinephrine (EPi), serotonin (5-HT), glutamate (GLU), and acetylcholine (ACh), also play a significant role (see Figure 2–1) (Everitt and Robbins 2005; Haile and Kosten 2001; Koob and Volkow 2010; Nestler 2005; M.J. Thomas et al. 2008; Weinshenker and Schroeder 2007). Moreover, in certain instances, syntheses of catecholamines (DA, NE, Epi) are dependent on each other. Altering enzymes essential for the normal production of these neurotransmitters at one point could affect levels of others downstream. For example, as shown in Figure 2–2, DA is converted to NE by the monoxygenase enzyme dopamine β-hydroxylase (DβH). Later in this chapter, we will see that disulfiram, a drug that shows efficacy in treating cocaine dependence, inhibits this enzyme. Inhibition of DβH, in turn, results in decreased NE levels, which is thought to underlie disulfiram's therapeutic effects.

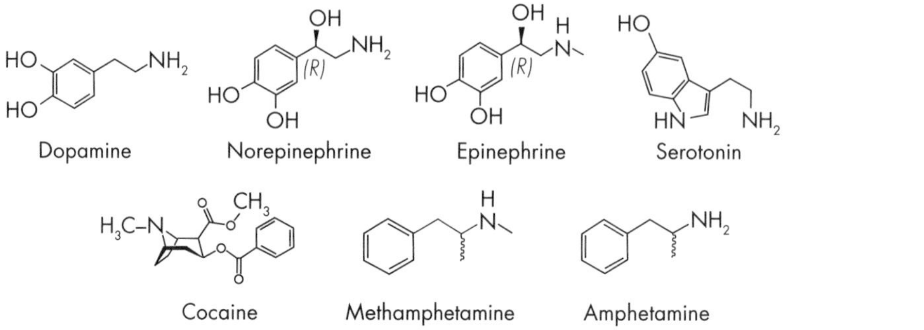

FIGURE 2–1. Chemical structures of stimulants and classical neuro-transmitters they alter.

Source. See Illustration Credits at conclusion of chapter.

DAergic cell bodies in the ventral tegmental area (VTA) and their projections to the prefrontal cortex (PFC) and nucleus accumbens (NAc) generally define the fundamental circuitry of the mesocorticolimbic system (see Figure 2–3). Other important brain structures associated with emotional memories, drug seeking, and drug taking include the amygdala, hippocampus, and hypothalamus (Everitt and Robbins 2005; A. Rocha and Kalivas 2010). Through different mechanisms all psychostimulants affect DA levels in the PFC and NAc, and lesions in these brain areas have been shown to alter their behavioral effects (Di Chiara and Imperato 1988; Pettit et al. 1984; Roberts and Koob 1982). GLU projections from the PFC to the NAc and VTA are also essential for psychostimulant action, as are NEergic innervation to these structures (Kalivas et al. 2003; Weinshenker and Schroeder 2007). Although oversimplified, this circuitry will serve as a model to help define the pharmacological action and the neural consequence of cocaine, METH, and AMPH.

A hypothetical scenario for a DA neuron and its target neuron is represented in Figure 2–4. In the simplest terms, DA released from vesicles into the synaptic cleft binds to a number of DA receptor subtypes, D_1-like (D_1, D_5) or D_2-like (D_2, D_3, D_4). These receptors are classified based on molecular and pharmacological characteristics. Activation of D_1-like receptors increases amounts of the second messenger cyclic adenosine 3′5′-monophosphate (cAMP) through stimulation of adenylate cyclase via G_s stimulatory G-proteins, whereas D_2 activation through G_i inhibitory G-proteins decreases the formation of cAMP. The formation of cAMP is dependent on adenylate cyclase, and cAMP is degraded by phosphodiesterase enzymes in the cytoplasm. Increased cAMP participates in a variety of intracellular processes that involve kinases such as protein kinase A (PKA) and G-protein receptor

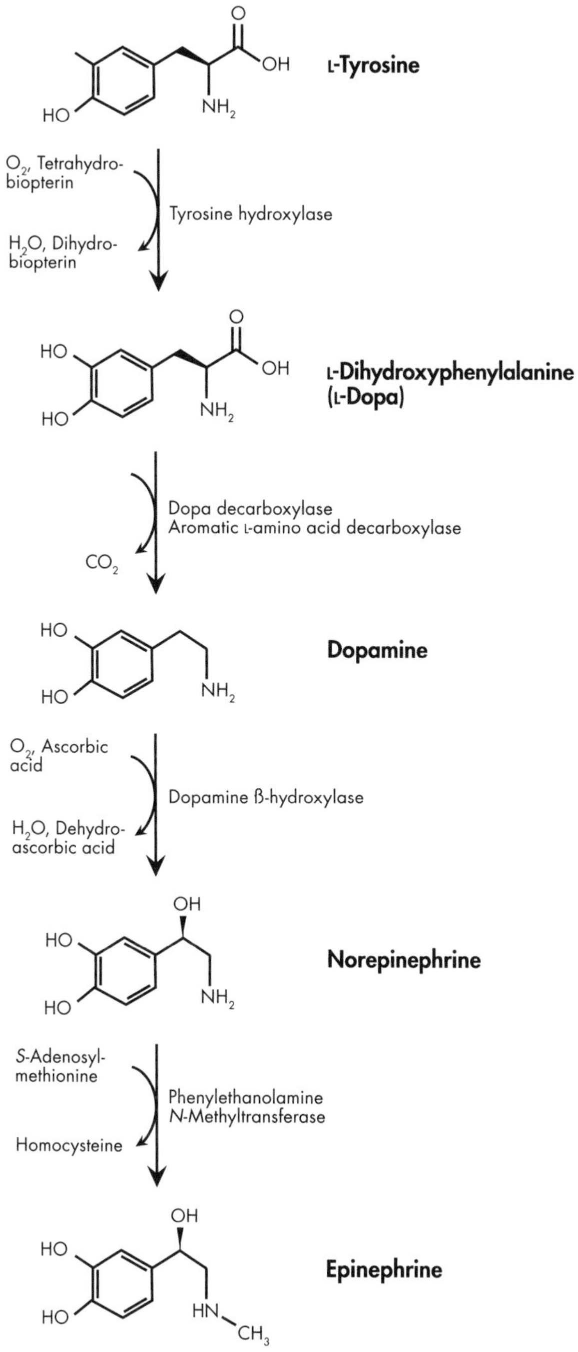

FIGURE 2–2. Essential steps in catecholamine biosynthesis.

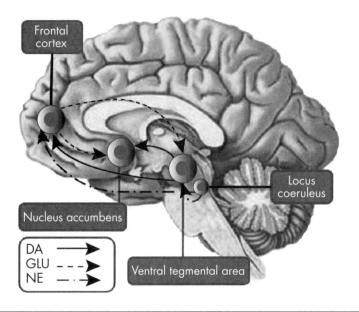

FIGURE 2–3.   Fundamental neurocircuitry governing the reinforcing effects of stimulants.

DA=dopamine; GLU=glutamate; NE=norepinephrine.

Source.   See Illustration Credits at conclusion of chapter.

kinase 3 (GRK3). PKA, for example, affects enzymes, phosphorylates receptors and channels, initiates the expression of various genes, and activates important transcription factors, such as cyclic adenosine monophosphate response-element binding protein (CREB) (Carlezon et al. 2005; Dinieri et al. 2009; Terwilliger et al. 1991). Important gene products implicated in psychostimulant effects include, among others, brain-derived neurotrophic factor (BDNF), cyclin-dependent kinase 5 (CDK5), nuclear factor kappa-B (NFkB), and AMPA glutamate receptor subtype-1 (GluR1), all of which mediate neuroplasticity related to aberrant reward learning in stimulant dependence (Ang et al. 2001; P. Chen and Chen 2005; Kim et al. 2005; Le Foll et al. 2005; Nestler 2002; Tsai 2007).

Neurotransmitter Release and Inactivation

A basic hypothetical DAergic synapse and the sequence of events presumed to occur between neurons are rendered in Figure 2–5. In general, following

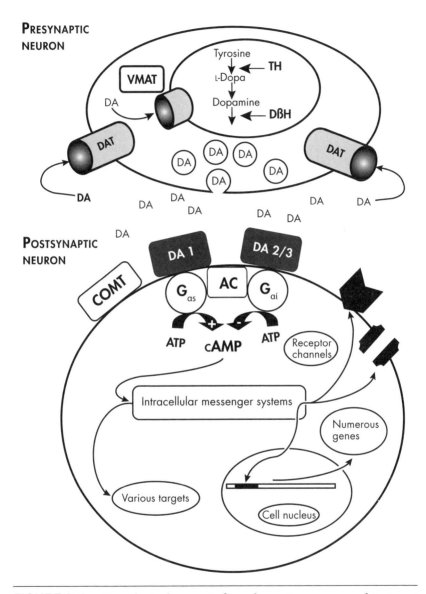

FIGURE 2–4.   Hypothetical scenario for a dopamine neuron and its target neuron.

AC=adenylate cyclase; ATP=adenosine triphosphate; cAMP=cyclic adenosine 3′5′-monophosphate; DA=dopamine; DAT=dopamine transporter; DβH=dopamine β-hydroxylase; $G_{\alpha i}$=inhibitory G-proteins; $G_{\alpha s}$=stimulatory G-proteins; TH=tyrosine hydroxylase; VMAT=vesicular monoamine transporter.

depolarization of the neuron, vesicles containing DA are mobilized and then fuse with the presynaptic membrane, releasing their contents into the synapse. Pharmacodynamic parameters then dictate the neurotransmitter's activation of presynaptic (autoreceptors) and postsynaptic DAergic receptor subtypes. Synaptic DA's action is then terminated by sequestration of the neurotransmitter back into the presynaptic neuron primarily through the DA transporter (DAT) (Glowinski and Iversen 1966; Snyder and Coyle 1969). Interestingly, DA is inactivated through reuptake by the NE transporter (NET) and by enzymatic conversion via catechol O-methyltransferase (COMT) in brain regions where DAT levels are low, such as in the PFC (Lewis et al. 2001; Morón et al. 2002).

Positive Subjective Effects of Stimulants

Studies have long associated DA neurotransmission with "euphoria" or the positive subjective effects elicited by psychostimulants. Controlled preclinical and clinical laboratory experiments have shown that psychostimulants possess potent reinforcing properties that are linked to positive subjective effects (Fischman and Schuster 1982; Haile and Kosten 2001; Hart et al. 2001; Newton et al. 2005a; Wachtel and de Wit 1999; Wise 1978). Activation of reward-related brain circuitry in humans (i.e., NAc or ventral striatum, PFC or frontal cortex) is associated with stimulant-induced euphoria (Völlm et al. 2004). A number of imaging studies in humans link DAT and D_2 receptor occupancy with cocaine and amphetamine-induced euphoria (Laruelle et al. 1998; Volkow et al. 1999b, 1999c). Interrupting DA neurotransmission with DA receptor antagonists (Newton et al. 2001; Sherer et al. 1989) or blocking DA metabolism (Alhassoon et al. 2001) partially attenuates these pleasurable subjective effects. The fact that disruption of DAergic action only partially diminishes the positive subjective effects of stimulants suggests other transmitter systems are involved. Indeed, recent data and reanalysis of older experiments in animals and humans show that NE plays a significant role in stimulant-induced effects (Weinshenker and Schroeder 2007). In fact, as will be detailed below, many promising medications for stimulant dependence target NE neurotransmission through a number of mechanisms (Baker et al. 2007; Carroll et al. 1998, 2004; De La Garza et al. 2010; Sofuoglu et al. 2009).

Animal Models of Human Drug Dependence

Early studies showed that drugs self-administered by humans were also self-administered by animals, suggesting that the motivational or reinforcing properties of these drugs are governed by primitive neurobiological sub-

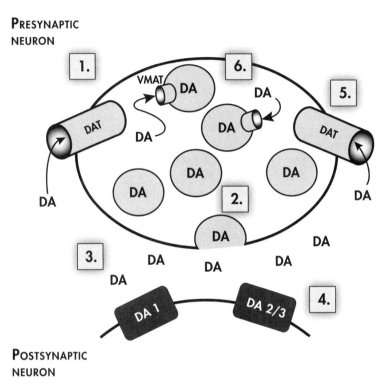

PRESYNAPTIC NEURON

POSTSYNAPTIC NEURON

1. DA neuron activation
2. Vesicular DA mobilized to terminals and released
3. Neurotransmitter in the synaptic cleft
4. Receptor subtypes activated
5. Inactivation of DA through the DAT
6. DA is sequestered into vesicles for repackaging

FIGURE 2–5. A basic hypothetical dopaminergic synapse and the sequence of events presumed to occur between neurons.

DA=dopamine; DAT=dopamine transporter; VMAT=vesicular monoamine transporter.

strates (Kornetsky and Esposito 1979; Olds and Milner 1954). An extensive literature describes experimental procedures used in animals that have also been applied to humans in a controlled laboratory setting (Comer et al. 2008). However, results from rodent and primate experimental paradigms often do not correlate with similar experiments in humans (Angarita et al. 2010). Nevertheless, important studies show that rodents can learn to control reward availability through instrumental learning, such as by pressing a lever ("operating" on something in the environment) to acquire an intra-venous injection of drug (Rescorla and Solomon 1967). In operant self-administration, environmental cues associated with a reinforcer help "stamp-in" a response (Bindra 1974). Extensive training can become habit-like and dissociated from the original reward (Balleine and Dickinson 1998). Cues paired with psychostimulants can then control behavior and increase re-sponding during extinction of self-administration of the drug (Panlilio et al. 1996). Increased responding at this stage likely reflects conditioned associ-ations of the context with drug effects, in which previously neutral stimuli acquire motivational value through incentive learning (Bindra 1974). Such stimuli increase responding to a primary reinforcer and act as reinforcers in their own right. This phenomenon may be related to relapse in humans that appears to reestablish and sustain addiction. Moreover, stimulants strengthen aberrant memory consolidation associated with the drug-taking process (White 1996) that, in theory, may promote drug craving and relapse in hu-mans (Berridge et al. 2009; Robinson and Berridge 1993). This part of the ad-diction process may overlap with normal learning mechanisms associated with neuroplastic changes. These long-lasting brain changes may contribute to the enduring nature of drug dependence (see next section).

Long-Lasting Drug Effects: Neuroplasticity

Although animal studies consistently showed that stimulants alter brain function, most of these changes reversed over time and thus could not ex-plain the unremitting relapsing that occurs in drug-dependent individuals. Eventually it was found, however, that enduring structural neural changes (i.e., neuroplasticity) occur in response to stimulants. These neuroplastic changes appeared to persist after drug exposure was discontinued, suggest-ing they may relate in some way to chronic relapsing in humans (Robinson and Kolb 2004). Indeed, long-lasting changes occur in discrete cytoskeletal proteins involved in the formation of new synapses or synaptogenesis Carl-isle and Kennedy 2005; Russo et al. 2010; Zuo et al. 2005). This finding was consistent with results showing stimulants enhance long-term potentiation (LTP), a cellular model of learning, in areas of the brain that govern their re-inforcing effects (Argilli et al. 2008). LTP is associated with the formation of new spines and enlargement of existing spines on neurons, whereas the op-posite process is associated with long-term depression (LTD) and both are el-emental to normal learning (Shen et al. 2009; M.J. Thomas et al. 2001). Altered DA and GLU neurotransmission appears to be essential to stimulant-induced effects on LTP/LTD (Argilli et al. 2008; Kalivas 2009; K.W. Lee et al. 2006). Whether preventing these changes in some way can play a role in the treatment of stimulant dependence in humans is not completely clear. However, pharmacotherapies that alter GLU neurotransmission, in particular, are an important focus of research (Pacchioni et al. 2009; Szumlinski et al. 2008).

Drugs of Abuse

Cocaine

Cocaine dependence remains a significant and persistent medical and social problem worldwide. In the United States, the National Survey on Drug Use and Health (U.S. Department of Health and Human Services 2009) notes that nearly 1.5 million Americans could be designated cocaine dependent. 2005 Drug Abuse Warning Network statistics show that about 800,000 emergency department visits were related to drug use (U.S. Department of Health and Human Services 2005) One-half million were cocaine related, whereas 100,000 were associated with METH abuse. Heart failure is common among the many adverse medical consequences of chronic cocaine use (Diercks et al. 2008). Medical debility secondary to major cardiovascular events and drug-related disease transmission related to cocaine use stress social and care management resources (Degenhardt et al. 2011). Indeed, cocaine is certainly the most deadly of all the street-acquired stimulants. Evidence-based ranking of each drug of abuse, using categories that included physical harm, dependence, and social harm as criteria, listed cocaine second only to the opioid heroin (Figure 2–6) (Nutt et al. 2007). Despite considerable effort to prevent transport of cocaine across borders, it is still readily available. For example, surface water sampling of a major river in a European country yielded the equivalent of approximately 1 kg of cocaine per day (Zuccato and Castiglioni 2009). Recognizing that this dangerous drug cannot be controlled, and that harsh penalties have not adequately deterred use, the recent emphasis on harm reduction and medical treatment may offer a better alternative to addressing the problem of drug dependence in general, and cocaine dependence in particular (Greenwald 2009; Mancini and Linhorst 2010).

"Über Coca": A Brief History of Cocaine

Cocaine was first extracted from the leaves of the coca plant (*Erythroxylon coca*) (Figure 2–7A) by Gaedcke in 1855. The extraction process was further refined a few years later by Niemann (1860). In contrast to the misuse and abuse of the relatively recently isolated compound cocaine, the coca leaf has been used among the Andean population in South America for over 3,000 years (Rivera et al. 2005). Archeological and historical evidence suggests the coca leaf was consumed as a daily tonic, used in a sacred religious rite, shared

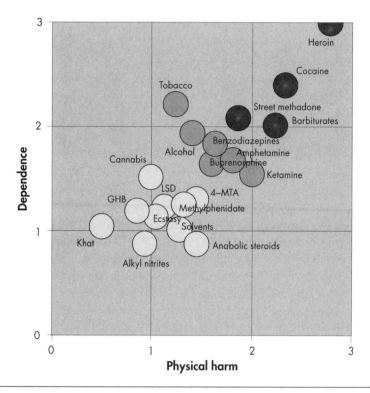

FIGURE 2–6.   Rational scale to assess the harm of drugs (mean physical harm and mean dependence).

GHB = γ-hydroxybutyric acid; LSD = lysergic acid diethylamide; 4-MTA = 4-methyl-thioamphetamine.

Source.   See Illustration Credits section at conclusion of chapter.

among people to enhance social bonding, and used medicinally. Today, the coca leaf is still chewed, but it is also ingested as a tea. The coca leaf is valued for its stimulant properties to stave off fatigue, as an anesthetic and an appetite suppressant, and to treat altitude sickness, among other illnesses (Indriati and Buikstra 2001). The leaves are sold in tea bags but also are contained in a variety of products readily available at grocery stores in Andean countries (i.e., Bolivia, Peru).

It is illegal in most countries to possess the coca plant or purified cocaine if it is not being used as indicated. However, this restriction does not apply to the Stepan Company (Maywood, New Jersey), which is the only company or institution that can legally import coca leaves (100 metric tons per year) and produce cocaine in the United States. Purified cocaine powder is, in turn, sold to Mallinckrodt Incorporated (St. Louis, Missouri), the only legal

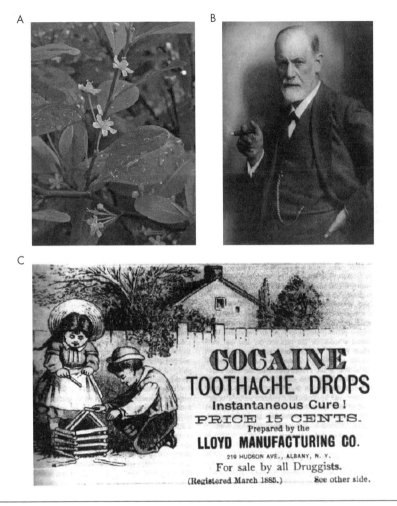

FIGURE 2–7. Images from the history of medicinal cocaine.

(A) Leaves of the coca plant (*Erythroxylon coca*). (B) Sigmund Freud (1922), who provided the first published detailed description of cocaine's potential medicinal properties in his landmark work "Über Coca," published in 1884. (C) Advertisement for an anesthetic patent medicine containing cocaine, 1865.

Source. See Illustration Credits at conclusion of chapter.

supplier of cocaine for the entire United States. Stepan Company provides "de-cocaineized" extracts from the leaves to the Coca-Cola and Red Bull companies as flavoring for their beverages (The Washington Times 2004). Coca-Cola drinks contained cocaine (4.5 mg per 6 oz) up until 1900, when it was excluded from the recipe (The New York Times 1988). Interestingly, Bolivia presently produces a drink called *Coca-Colla* that uses the coca leaf as its base ingredient. This beverage presumably is similar to the recipe the U.S. Coca-Cola company abandoned in the early twentieth century (lanacion.com 2010).

Sigmund Freud, the father of psychoanalysis (Figure 2–7B), provided the first published detailed description of cocaine's potential medicinal properties (Shaffer 1984). In his landmark work "Über Coca," published in 1884, Freud exhausted all known resources, noting the history and pharmacology of the coca leaf, including experiments on animals and humans. Among the human experiments mentioned, Freud described his own experiences, having ingested cocaine at least 12 times with positive effects. Cocaine appeared to be a viable treatment for "diverse kinds of psychic debility," including alcohol and morphine dependence (Freud and Byck 1975). It was cocaine's use in surgical ophthalmology as a topical anesthetic, however, that pushed the drug to the top of the pharmacological armamentarium (Goldberg 1984) (Figure 2–7C). Unfortunately, it became readily apparent that cocaine in its purified form was highly addictive, and cocaine eventually fell out of favor, nearly destroying Freud's reputation in the process (Shaffer 1984).

Pharmacology and Pharmacokinetics

Cocaine exists in primarily two forms. The pure salt form, cocaine hydrochloride, is a white powder (Figure 2–8), whereas its base form (i.e., freebase) is typically white to light brown, depending on impurities. Cocaine hydrochloride is water soluble and thus can be administered intravenously. The freebase crystalline form of cocaine, or "crack," is insoluble in water and is usually smoked. The term *crack* is derived from the audible crackling noise produced when cocaine in this form is smoked.

Characteristic street forms of cocaine contain adulterants used to dilute the drug but increase volume for subsequent sales. Common adulterants include sugar, baking soda, and anesthetics such as lidocaine and benzocaine (Fucci and De Giovanni 1998; McKinney et al. 1992). Street cocaine may also contain other stimulants, such as caffeine and/or medications such as diltiazem, acetaminophen, hydroxyzine, and an analgesic known to be carcinogenic, phenacetin (Brunt et al. 2009; Evrard et al. 2010; Fucci and De Giovanni 1998). More problematic is the recent finding that nearly 70% of seized cocaine entering the United States is adulterated with the agranulocytosis-inducing anthelmintic drug levamisole, which is responsible for numerous hospitalizations and deaths (Centers for Disease Control and Prevention 2009; Czuchlewski et al. 2010). Why this particular medication is so prevalently used as an adulterant to dilute cocaine powder is an interesting and pressing question from a pharmacological viewpoint.

Cocaine is primarily metabolized by the liver and plasma cholinesterases to the inactive water-soluble metabolites benzoylecgonine and ecgonine

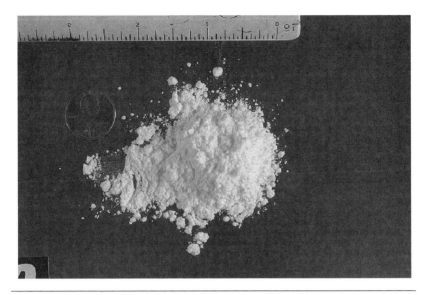

FIGURE 2–8.   Cocaine hydrochloride, the salt form of cocaine.
Source.   See Illustration Credits at conclusion of chapter.

methyl ester. These metabolites are then excreted in the urine and represent approximately 90% of the original cocaine dose, but a small remaining percentage is excreted as intact parent compound (Jatlow 1988; Van Dyke et al. 1977). Interestingly, hepatic N-demethylated cocaine yields a very small percentage of norcocaine, a pharmacologically active metabolite (Hawks et al. 1974). Numerous other minor inactive metabolites are also produced (Kolbrich et al. 2006).

The route of administration determines the time at which cocaine is detected in blood. Table 2–2 summarizes systemic bioavailability of cocaine via various routes and in different formulations. As noted, the oral smoking route results in rapid entry of cocaine into systemic circulation. Indeed, the pharmacokinetics of smoked cocaine—which are similar to those of intravenously administered cocaine—underlie its potent reinforcing and addictive characteristics. That is, plasma concentrations of cocaine are directly correlated to its physiological and subjective effects (Javaid et al. 1978; Newton et al. 2005a). The rapidity with which the freebase formulation enters systemic circulation is a key element to cocaine's addictive potency. This feature is consistent with findings from human imaging studies, which demonstrated that the more quickly an addictive drug enters systemic circulation, the faster it crosses the blood-brain barrier, and the higher the abuse liability (Fowler et al. 2008; Reed et al. 2009; Volkow et al. 2000).

TABLE 2–2. Pharmacokinetic profile of different routes of cocaine administration

Drug	Route	Dose	N	Bio-availability	T_{max} (min)	C_{max} (ng/mL)	$t_{1/2}$ (min)	Reference
Cocaine	IV	25 mg	6	–	37	230	89	Cone 1995
	IN	32 mg	6	94%		63	–	
	Oral	42 mg	5	70%		227	82	
	IV	32 mg	3–10	–	4	260	38	Isenschmid et al. 1992
	Oral	50 mg	3–10	–	4	220	39	
	IV	23 mg	4	–	30	180	78	Jeffcoat et al. 1989
	IN	106 mg	4	80%		220	–	
	Oral	50 mg	6	60%		203	58	
	IV	40 mg	5	–	–		37	Cone et al. 1988
	IV	0.23–0.29 mg/kg	6	–	–	–	87	Cook et al. 1985
	Oral	0.4–0.6 mg/kg	6	57%			88	
	IV	32 mg	4	–	–		41	Javaid et al. 1978, 1983
	IN	64 mg	4		30	115	42	
	IN	96 mg	4		–		84	
	IN	64 mg	–		37	67	–	
	IN	0.19–2.0 mg/kg (10% solution)	7	25%	66	44.5	75	Wilkinson et al. 1980
	Oral	2–3 mg/kg	4	–	–	–	48	

TABLE 2–2. Pharmacokinetic profile of different routes of cocaine administration *(continued)*

Drug	Route	Dose	N	Bio-availability	T_{max} (min)	C_{max} (ng/mL)	$t_{1/2}$ (min)	Reference
	IV	32 mg	5	–			48	Chow et al. 1985
	IV	1 mg/kg	–	60%	–	–	38	Barnett et al. 1981
	IV	3 mg/kg					87	
	IN	96 mg					90	
	IN	2 mg/kg					74	
	IN	1.5 mg/kg	9	–	60	308	–	Van Dyke et al. 1976, 1978
	IN	2 mg/kg	4	–	60	160	78	
	Oral	2 mg/kg	4	–	60	209	54	

Note. IN=intranasal; IV=intravenous; Oral=smoked or liquid solution where indicated.

Preclinical Behavioral Pharmacology

Assessing cocaine's effects in animal models of human drug dependence has been essential in determining its central pharmacological action. Cocaine induces a wide array of behavioral effects in animals, as shown by numerous behavioral models. For example, acute administration of low to moderate doses stimulates movement usually measured as locomotor activity (Wise and Bozarth 1987). However, high doses of cocaine decrease locomotion by inducing stereotyped behaviors (e.g., sniffing, chewing, rearing) that impede movement (Barr et al. 1983). These behavioral effects can increase (sensitize) with repeated drug dosing over time, so that low doses provoke behavior originally associated with high doses of the drug (Ellinwood and Balster 1974; Robinson and Berridge 1993; Wise and Bozarth 1987). Some researchers hypothesize that drug craving in humans may be a type of sensitization reflecting unconscious, unconditioned, and conditioned processes that contributes to continued drug seeking and drug taking (Robinson and Berridge 1993). For example, if repeated drug administrations are paired with exposure to a specific context, such as a novel locomotor apparatus, exposure to that context can provoke a greater behavioral response (Robinson and Berridge 1993; Stewart et al. 1984). It is likely that the unconditioned and context-conditioning effects of repeated cocaine exposure reflect different but interconnected neural circuits. In addition, neural circuits that contribute to the development of locomotor sensitization to cocaine differ from those that contribute to its expression (Vanderschuren and Kalivas 2000). Similarly, the development and expression of cocaine place conditioning may also reflect different neuropharmacological mechanisms (Spyraki et al. 1982).

Cocaine can modify behavior by acting as a cue or discriminative stimulus that can elicit a specific behavioral response (Broadbent et al. 1995; Colpaert et al. 1976; Katz et al. 1991; Kleven et al. 1990; McKenna and Ho 1980). That is, cocaine administered via injection can, for example, signal to the animal that pressing on a lever paired with cocaine will result in a food pellet, whereas pressing on a saline-paired lever will not. Studies using this behavioral paradigm demonstrate that the cocaine discriminative stimulus is pharmacologically specific and generalizes to other compounds that have similar pharmacological actions, such as DA releasers (e.g., amphetamine) or DA reuptake inhibitors (C.D. Cook et al. 2002). In contrast, animals' ability to learn to discriminate cocaine shows that drugs that are not in the same class as cocaine (i.e., are not psychostimulants) do not generalize to compounds with dissimilar pharmacological actions or to those in a different drug class (e.g., pentobarbital). The degree to which the discriminative stimulus effects of a substance generalize to a known drug of abuse is thought to be a good predictor of abuse liability (Solinas et al. 2006). There is a good deal of concordance between the discriminative stimulus effects and subjective effects of drugs in humans (Johanson et al. 2006; Kamien et al. 1993). Drugs that act on the DA, NE, and GLU systems significantly affect cocaine's discriminative stimulus in animals and humans (B. Lee et al. 2005; Lile et al. 2010; Negus et al. 2007; Sinnott et al. 1999).

Psychostimulants, such as cocaine, ingested by humans are also self-administered by animals (Seevers and Schuster 1967). Thus, the drug self-administration behavioral paradigm in animals would apparently possess excellent face validity as an animal model of drug addiction in humans (Deroche-Gamonet et al. 2004; Vanderschuren and Everitt 2004). Like the dependent human in procuring drug, the animal must perform a voluntary response (e.g., lever-pressing in an operant chamber) to receive the drug intravenously or orally (Caine and Koob 1993; Comer et al. 2008). In this paradigm, drugs that increase the likelihood that the behavior preceding the drug infusion will occur again are said to serve as reinforcers or to be reinforcing (Pickens et al. 1968; Schuster and Thompson 1969). The fact that numerous psychoactive drugs self-administered by humans also serve as reinforcers in animals strongly suggests that the drug self-administration paradigm may also serve to predict abuse liability of possible pharmacotherapies (Collins et al. 1984; Comer et al. 2008).

Different drug self-administration paradigms can model certain aspects of addiction, such as vulnerability, maintenance, craving, compulsiveness, and relapse. For example, acquisition of drug self-administration behavior may model vulnerability to addiction (Deminiere et al. 1989). Drug "craving" or drug "seeking" may be modeled by replacing the drug with saline and measuring time to extinguish self-administration behavior or persistence of responding (Markou et al. 1993). Replacing the drug with saline extinguishes cocaine self-administration behavior. This behavior can be reestablished with noncontingent cocaine infusions, conditioned cues, and foot-shock stress even though cocaine is not available (Ahmed and Koob 1997; Erb et al. 1996; Piazza and LeMoal 1998). These animal models of "relapse" (de Wit and Stewart 1981; Markou et al. 1993) may be applicable to humans, since cocaine-dependent individuals report craving as one of many reasons they tend to relapse (Gawin and Kleber 1986). Further research is needed to establish the predictive validity of these relapse models as they apply to humans, however (Katz and Higgins 2003).

Clinical Behavioral Pharmacology

One of the many goals of human laboratory research has been to develop a pharmacotherapy for cocaine dependence. Much scientific information regarding cocaine's pharmacological and physiological effects has been meticulously collected, yet no medication has gained an indication for this dependency. This is likely because of cocaine's complex central effects on numerous neurotransmitter systems and their receptors and its potent reinforcing properties. Indeed, regardless of what route, humans dose-dependently self-administer cocaine under controlled laboratory conditions (Comer et al. 2008; Fischman et al. 1976; Foltin et al. 2003; Muntaner et al. 1989; Newton et al. 2005a; Stoops et al. 2010). However, when given a choice, cocaine-dependent volunteers in one study preferred the smoking route (Foltin and Fischman 1992). The reason for this choice in route is intriguing and may be more related to the rapid and potent euphoric effects of freebase ("crack") cocaine. For example, in one pharmacokinetic study assessing cocaine, volunteers rated the subjective effects of cumulative smoking doses (0, 25, and 50 mg) greater than those of intravenously administered cocaine (0, 16, and 32 mg). Although both smoked and intravenously administered cocaine result in similar systemic concentrations and produce equal effects on cardiovascular measures, the potency of smoked cocaine doses was much less than that for the intravenous doses. Yet, volunteers' subjective ratings were greater for smoked cocaine than for intravenous cocaine (Foltin and Fischman 1991). Again, the rapidity at which this formulation enters arterial systemic circulation (15 seconds vs. 4 minutes) may be why smoking cocaine is such a common route of self-administration (Evans et al. 1996).

Unlike the sensitization to the behavioral effects of cocaine seen in animals, tolerance quickly develops to the cardiovascular and subjective effects produced by cocaine in humans (Foltin and Fischman 1991; Foltin and Haney 2004; Reed et al. 2009; Ward et al. 1997a, 1997b). The neurochemical mechanisms that underlie tolerance to cocaine's effects are not known. Recent evidence suggests, however, that chronic cocaine use renders the DAT insensitive to cocaine's effects, whereas AMPH, which is a substrate for the DAT (see below), maintains its potent effects on this transporter (Ferris et al. 2011). The fact that AMPH remains active at the DAT after chronic cocaine treatment supports a growing literature that chronic treatment with immediate-release and sustained-release (SR) AMPH and METH medications that are indicated to treat attention-deficit/hyperactivity disorder (ADHD) in adolescents and adults may be used as pharmacotherapies for cocaine dependence. Indeed, chronic dosing with therapeutic formulations of AMPH and METH lessens the subjective effects of cocaine and decreases cocaine use in laboratory and clinical outpatient trials, respectively (Grabowski et al. 2001; Herin et al. 2010; Mooney et al. 2009; Rush et al. 2009, 2010; Shearer et al. 2003).

Effects on Dopamine Neurotransmission

Natural rewards such as food (Wang et al. 2006) and drugs of abuse (including cocaine) activate the mesocorticolimbic DA system (Wise and Rompre

1989). Cocaine has numerous effects on physiology and neurochemistry; however, it is well established that the primary mechanism that significantly contributes to its potent reinforcing effects is DA reuptake inhibition (Harris and Baldessarini 1973). This action, in turn, increases synaptic DA to supraphysiological levels (Pettit and Justice 1989) (Figure 2–9). Clear evidence shows that cocaine's reinforcing properties are linked to its ability to increase synaptic DA by binding to the DAT (Ritz et al. 1987). Indeed, molecularly engineering the DAT in such a way that it is insensitive to cocaine abolishes its potent reinforcing effects (Thomsen et al. 2009). DATs inserted into the neuronal membrane translocate DA back inside the cell via a concentration gradient negating DA action on pre- and postsynaptic receptors. DA may then be degraded by the enzyme monoamine oxidase or sequestered back into synaptic vesicles by vesicular monoamine transporter–2 (VMAT-2). Acute exposure to cocaine increases DAT insertion into the membrane to sequester and negate supraphysiological concentrations of DA (Glowinski and Iversen 1966; Snyder and Coyle 1969). Similarly, cocaine triggers redistribution of VMAT-2 into synaptic vesicles (Riddle et al. 2002) (Figure 2–9).

Because one of cocaine's primary mechanisms of action is to alter DA levels, research aimed at identifying a therapeutic drug for cocaine dependence has focused on either blocking postsynaptic DA receptor subtypes or targeting presynaptic autoreceptors that regulate DA release. Unfortunately, however, such approaches have not been fruitful. In contrast, medications that have the opposite mechanism of action—that stimulate DA receptors and increase DA levels—show some efficacy for cocaine dependence (Castells et al. 2010; Pérez-Mañá et al. 2011). Moreover, recent research focused on neurotransmitter systems *other* than DA has yielded significant advances in defining cocaine's addictive action on brain neurochemistry as it relates to medication development (Weinshenker and Schroeder 2007). Most important is the finding that promising medications for cocaine dependence, such as SR formulations of AMPH and METH, more potently alter NE neurotransmission in various ways than they do DA neurotransmission (Table 2–3) (Rothman et al. 2001). The fact that these medications alter NE neurotransmission in such a profound manner suggests that affecting NE neurotransmission may be a better therapeutic strategy for cocaine dependence.

Effects on Norepinephrine Neurotransmission

Similar to its action on DA, cocaine also blocks 5-HT and NE reuptake, elevating synaptic levels of these neurotransmitters. Studies suggest that 5-HT contributes to some behavioral effects produced by cocaine, although NE appears to play a more important role (K.A. Cunningham et al. 2010; Filip et al. 2010; B.A. Rocha et al. 1998). Genetically altering NE production in animals, or administering drugs that target NE by facilitating release, blocking

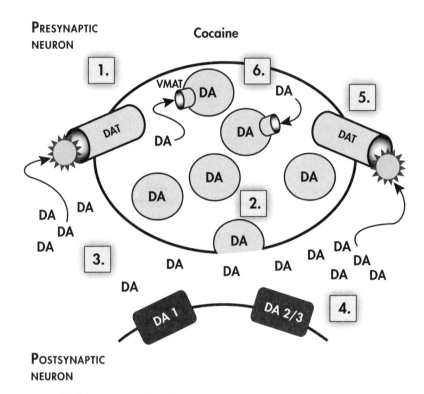

1. DA neuron activation
2. Vesicular DA mobilized to terminals and released
3. Cocaine increases neurotransmitter in the synaptic cleft
4. Receptor subtypes activated
5. Cocaine prevents the inactivation of DA by blocking the DAT
6. DA is repackaged into vesicles by way of the VMAT

FIGURE 2–9.　Impact of cocaine at the dopaminergic synapse related to its potent reinforcing effects.

DA=dopamine; DAT=dopamine transporter; VMAT=vesicular monoamine transporter.

its synthesis, or blocking specific receptor subtypes, significantly alters cocaine's effects (Baker et al. 2007; Carroll et al. 2004; Haile et al. 2003; Hameedi et al. 1995; Herin et al. 2010; Oliveto et al. 2011; Petrakis et al. 2000; Schroeder et al. 2010; Weinshenker and Schroeder 2007). The exact role of NE in mediating psychostimulant behavioral and subjective effects in humans is unknown. The fact that circuitry crucial to cocaine's reinforcement is apparently under NE control suggests possible interactions with central DA (see Figure 2–3). For example, NEergic neurons project to forebrain

TABLE 2–3. Release and uptake inhibition of drugs and neurotransmitters

Drug	NE release IC50 (nM)	NE uptake Ki (nM)	5-HT release IC50 (nM)	5-HT uptake Ki (nM)	DA release IC50 (nM)	DA uptake Ki (nM)
Cocaine	>10,000	779±30	>10,000	304±10	>10,000	478±25
d-Amphetamine	7.07±0.9	38.9±1.8	1,765±94	3,830±17	24.8±3.5	34±60
l-Methamphetamine	28.5±2.5	234±14	4,640±24	14,000±64	416±20	4,840±17
d-Methamphetamine	12.3±0.7	48±5.1	736±45	2,137±98	24.5±2.1	114±11
MDMA	77.4±3.4	462±18	56.6±2.1	238±13	376±16	1,572±59
Dopamine	66.2±5.4	40.3±4.4	>10,000	6,489±20	86.9±9.7	38.3±1.6
Norepinephrine	164±13	63.9±1.6	>10,000	>50,000	869±51	357±27
Serotonin	>10,000	3,013±26	44.4±5.3	16.7±0.9	>10,000	2,703±79

Note.   DA=dopamine; 5-HT=5-hydroxytryptamine (serotonin); MDMA=3,4-methylenedioxymethamphetamine; NE=norepinephrine.
Source.   Matecka et al. 1996; Rothman and Baumann 2006; Rothman et al. 1993, 2001.

structures, where they interact with DA in the NAc and PFC (Morrison et al. 1981; Shi et al. 2000; Swanson and Hartman 1975). NE terminals can take up and release DA in the PFC, and is released with NE when locus coeruleus NE cell bodies are stimulated (Devoto et al. 2001, 2005). Evidence also suggests that DA can stimulate NE/EPi receptors. It is well known that DA is an agonist in the periphery and activates α-adrenergic receptors on vasculature, causing vasoconstriction, and β-adrenergic receptors on the heart, stimulating the organ, having both inotropic and chronotropic effects. In fact, DA and its derivative dobutamine are drugs of choice to treat severe shock. That DA and NE may cross-talk centrally is logical and likely. Indeed, evidence suggests that DA, not NE, is the endogenous agonist at α_{2C}-adrenergic receptors in the striatum (W. Zhang and Ordway 2003; W. Zhang et al. 1999).

More specific to psychostimulants, NE activation of cortical α_1-adrenergic receptors increases NAc DA and augments stimulant-induced locomotor activity, both of which are blocked by intra-PFC injections of the α_1 antagonist prazosin (Blanc et al. 1994; Darracq et al. 1998; Drouin et al. 2002). Further, genetically ablated α_{1B}-adrenergic receptor mice show decreased stimulant-induced activity (Drouin et al. 2002). NE affects metabotropic GLU receptors that normally inhibit DA cells, and stimulants counteract this effect, thereby increasing DA neurotransmission that is α_1 receptor–dependent (Paladini et al. 2001). Thus, α_1-adrenergic receptors may mediate cocaine's effects by increasing DA through a PFC-NAc GLUergic circuit (Miner et al. 2003; Sesack et al. 2003). Interestingly, this neural circuit may be critical in drug-seeking behaviors because systemically administered prazosin reduces cocaine-induced reinstatement of cocaine self-administration and prevents the enhancement of cocaine self-administration in animals with prior drug exposure (Kalivas and McFarland 2003; X. Y. Zhang and Kosten 2005, 2007).

Effects on Glutamate Neurotransmission

As shown for DA and NE, studies indicate GLU neurotransmission also plays a significant role in drug reward and reinforcement (Figure 2–3) and may offer still another therapeutic target for the treatment of cocaine dependence (Bowers et al. 2010; Kalivas 2009; Schmidt and Pierce 2010). GLU is the most ubiquitous excitatory neurotransmitter in the brain and is essential for a myriad of processes, including neuroplasticity linked to long-term potentiation, long-term depression, extinction, and reward-related learning (B. T. Chen et al. 2008; Knackstedt et al. 2010; Novak et al. 2010; Sarti et al. 2007; Shen et al. 2009). Recent preclinical studies report that GLU projections from the PFC to the NAc are critical for cue-induced, stress-induced, and cocaine-primed reinstatement of previously extinguished cocaine self-administration behavior in animals (Bäckström and Hyytiä 2007; Cornish and Kalivas 2000; Knackstedt et al. 2010; Ping et al. 2008). AMPA (ionotropic glutamate α-amino-3-hydroxy-5-methyl-4-isoxazolepropionic acid) infused into the NAc induces reinstatement of cocaine self-administration, whereas translational blockade by antisense oligonucleotides aimed at the GluR1 AMPA receptor subtype blocks this behavior (Ping et al. 2008). The AMPA GLU receptors have consistently been implicated in the behavioral effects of psychostimulants (Bowers et al. 2010; Carlezon and Nestler 2002; Knackstedt et al. 2010). For example, repeated cocaine exposure increases GluR1 levels in the VTA (Fitzgerald et al. 1996). Increasing CREB in the VTA upregulates GluR1, whereas ablating CREB in a manner that blocks endogenous levels of CREB decreases GluR1 levels (Olson et al. 2005). The presynaptic autoreceptors metabotropic mGluR2/3, which regulate the release of GLU when stimulated, can attenuate cocaine- and cue-induced reinstatement (Adewale et al. 2006; Anwyl 1999). Similarly, GLU receptor antagonist ligands aimed at postsynaptic mGluR5 receptors equally block cue-induced cocaine reinstatement (Bäckström and Hyytiä 2006; Iso et al. 2006). Taken together, these findings highlight an ever-expanding role of GLU receptor subtypes in cocaine's behavioral effects and may offer clues to possible pharmacotherapeutic targets for cocaine dependence.

Until recently, the lack of ligands to specific GLU receptor subtypes and the innate complexity of this neurotransmitter system have hampered in-depth study of GLU's role in psychostimulant dependence and subsequent development of viable pharmacotherapies. Although it is presently unknown whether GLU neurotransmission is compromised in cocaine-dependent individuals, GLU dysregulation is readily induced by psychostimulants in animals. For example, NAc GLU levels are maintained by the glial cystine-glutamate antiporter—which exchanges cystine molecules one-to-one with GLU—and this antiporter is downregulated following exposure to cocaine. Cocaine's action compromises the antiporter, in turn, leading to low levels of basal GLU (Baker et al. 2002, 2003). Importantly, basal levels of GLU in the NAc mediate reinstatement of cocaine self-administration, which may relate to relapse in humans (Baker et al. 2003; Kau et al. 2008). One way to restore accumbal GLU levels and neurotransmitter tone is with the cystine prodrug N-acetylcysteine. N-Acetylcysteine blocks cocaine reinstatement and appears to reengage mGluR2/3 autoreceptors that control GLU release (Baker et al. 2003; Moran et al. 2005). N-Acetylcysteine also reverses many cocaine-induced effects on proteins involved in neuroplasticity that have been shown to be important in animal models of relapse (Madayag et al. 2007; Moussawi et al. 2009). Clinical studies in humans generally support N-acetylcysteine's efficacy for cocaine dependence, confirming preclinical findings. In short, N-acetylcysteine appears to block some of cocaine's subjective effects and dampen reactivity to drug cues that elicit craving (LaRowe et al. 2006, 2007;

Mardikian et al. 2007). Larger randomized double-blind placebo-controlled trials are needed, however, to confirm these promising preliminary findings.

Neural Deficiencies in Cocaine Dependence: Pharmacotherapeutic Targets

Understanding neurochemical abnormalities in cocaine-dependent individuals may help guide medication development. Indeed, several abnormalities localized primarily in structures that compose the mesocorticolimbic system and striatum have been clearly identified. Figure 2–10 represents a hypothetical neural synapse with a presynaptic DAergic neuron and a postsynaptic neuron expressing DAergic receptors. Normally, DA is synthesized from the precursor DOPA by dopa-decarboxylase (Figure 2–10A[1]), packaged into vesicles and released upon depolarization of the neuron (Figure 2–10A[2]). Vesicular DA released into the synaptic cleft (Figure 2–10A[3]) stimulates DAergic receptors of various subtypes (Figure 2–10A[4]) and subsequently is inactivated through reuptake by the DAT (Figure 2–10A[5]). In certain brain areas, the NET can also sequester and thereby inactivate DA in addition to NE. Imaging studies reveal that cocaine-dependent individuals exhibit significant abnormalities in DAergic neurotransmission in ventral and dorsal striatum and cortical brain areas (Volkow et al. 2010). These abnormalities include decreased DA synthesis (Figure 2–10B[1]) (Wu et al. 1997), reduced endogenous DA levels (Figure 2–10B[2]) (Martinez et al. 2009), blunted stimulant-induced DA release (Figure 2–10B[3]) (Martinez et al. 2007), reduced D_2/D_3 receptor levels (Figure 2–10B[4]) (Martinez et al. 2004, 2009; Volkow et al. 1993), and increased DAT (Crits-Christoph et al. 2008) and cortical NET levels (Ding et al. 2010). Some of these abnormalities are likely not due to chronic cocaine use per se, since these deficits are not fully reversed on prolonged withdrawal. Rather, abnormalities in DA neurotransmission in cocaine-dependent individuals may indeed represent a vulnerable neurobiological phenotype.

Some researchers attempting to address the lack of pharmacotherapeutics for cocaine dependence have adopted an agonist-like substitution approach similar to that used with methadone and buprenorphine for opioid dependence (Herin et al. 2010). Modafinil is a wake-promoting medication indicated for narcolepsy and shift-work somnolence (Jasinski and Kovacevi-Ristanovi 2000). Modafinil's mechanism of action is not fully understood, but it appears to increase DA/NE levels by blocking reuptake, and it promotes GLU neurotransmission (Ferraro et al. 1997; Madras et al. 2006). Modafinil was shown to have discriminative stimulus effects similar to those of cocaine in animals (Gold and Balster 1996); however, this finding was not replicated in a human study (Rush et al. 2002). Similarly, although its DAT binding is similar to cocaine's in humans, modafinil is not readily self-administered by

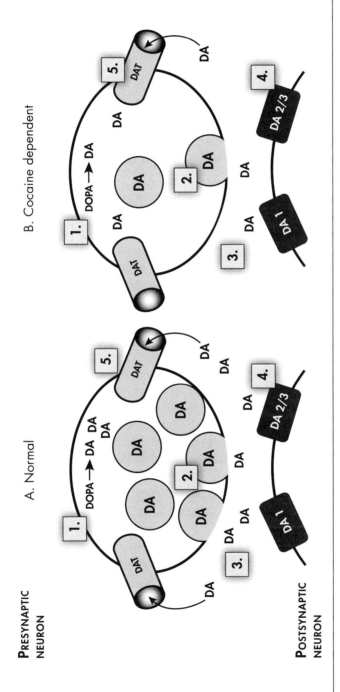

FIGURE 2–10. Hypothetical neural synapse (with a presynaptic dopaminergic neuron and a postsynaptic neuron expressing dopaminergic receptors) in (A) normal and (B) cocaine-dependent individuals, illustrating abnormalities localized primarily in structures that compose the mesocorticolimbic system.

DA=dopamine; DAT=dopamine transporter.

cocaine-dependent individuals (Volkow et al. 2009; Vosburg et al. 2010). In fact, studies demonstrate that modafinil *decreases* cocaine use and *blocks* the subjective effects of cocaine administered in the laboratory (Dackis et al. 2003, 2005; Hart et al. 2008b). However, modafinil does not appear to be efficacious in cocaine-dependent individuals who also meet criteria for alcohol dependence (Anderson et al. 2009).

Other stimulant-like medications, such as SR formulations of AMPH and METH, reduce cocaine's subjective effects and cocaine use in dependent individuals. The mechanisms that underlie these effects are unknown but could involve reversal of some abnormalities seen in DAergic neurotransmission mentioned earlier. At doses used to treat diseases such as ADHD, refractory obesity, and narcolepsy, SR-AMPH and SR-METH both increase DAergic synthesis and neurotransmitter release in striatum and increase activity in cortical areas known to be involved in working memory and impulse control, both of which are compromised in cocaine-dependent individuals (Martinez et al. 2004, 2007, 2009; Narendran et al. 2009). SR-AMPH and SR-METH also alter the DAT and induce DA efflux, further increasing DA (Martinez et al. 2007; Sulzer et al. 2005). Chronic treatment with stimulant-like medications may increase basal DAergic tone in DA-depleted cocaine-dependent individuals. However, chronic treatment with SR stimulants also results in tolerance to subsequent pharmacological challenges with stimulants such as cocaine, suggesting that tolerance may be another mechanism involved in SR stimulant therapeutic action (Chiodo et al. 2008; Negus and Mello 2003; Peltier et al. 1996; Rush et al. 2009).

The accumulating experimental evidence reviewed above indicates that NE is associated with the euphoric effects of cocaine and more closely related to craving that leads to relapse to cocaine use after a period of abstinence (Weinshenker and Schroeder 2007). This should not be surprising, since locus coeruleus NEergic cell bodies project diffusely throughout the human brain innervating the VTA, NAc, and other areas implicated in cocaine's effects (Smythies 2005). Activation of locus coeruleus neurons increases VTA DA neuronal firing (Lategan et al. 1990). NE in the PFC also increases VTA DA activity that is dose dependent (Blanc et al. 1994). Whereas acute AMPH administration inhibits DA neurons in the VTA, chronic treatment is associated with the opposite effect of excitation (Kamata and Rebec 1984). Chronic AMPH-induced excitation in the VTA may relate to "tolerance" to the reinforcing effects of cocaine observed in a number of preclinical studies and may explain some of the beneficial effects of these stimulants for cocaine dependence. However, because of the innate abuse-liability associated with stimulant drugs, alternative nonstimulant medications such as DA precursors (Mooney et al. 2007; Schmitz et al. 2008), stimulant prodrugs with delayed absorption (Jasinski and Krishnan 2009), or anorectic medications with a proven track record of safety (Rothman et al. 2008) may be a better therapeutic option.

Methamphetamine and Amphetamine

The search for efficacious medications to treat METH and AMPH dependence has proved difficult (Karila et al. 2010). Recent "epidemics" in the United States and abroad have focused more attention than ever on the drugs' powerful addictive properties, ease of production, availability, and systemic and central toxic effects. As described in Chapter 1 ("Epidemiology and Psychiatric Comorbidity"), monitoring the purchase and importation of precursor chemicals has likely decreased the previously sharp upward trends of METH availability and use (J.K. Cunningham et al. 2009; Drug Enforcement Administration 2008). Unfortunately, this has led to the use of inferior alternate synthesis methods that often yield a product with very toxic adulterants and synthetic by-products. Indeed, after new laws were initiated, prices for METH increased dramatically while purity decreased from 90% to 20% (Dobkin and Nicosia 2009).

Intimate Drug History

METH and AMPH are inextricably linked by their chemical structures, mechanism of action, and historical use (Anglin et al. 2000; Haile 2007; Rasmussen 2008). These drugs are usually synthesized from simple precursor chemicals, although small amounts have been reported to be present naturally in plants (Clement et al. 1997, 1998). AMPH was originally synthesized by the German chemist Lazar Edeleanu in 1887. Independent of Edeleanu's discovery, Gordon Alles in 1927 again synthesized the drug (known then as beta-phenyl-isopropylamine) and assessed its physiological effects, publishing the results in the 1930s and patenting use of the oral salt form (Alles 1933; Piness et al. 1930). Smith, Kline, and French introduced the Benzedrine Inhaler, which contained 325 mg of AMPH (a racemic mixture of *d*- and *l*-AMPH; the *d* isomer is sevenfold more potent that the *l* isomer). The Benzadrine Inhaler was first sold over the counter in the early 1930s for the treatment of asthma. Endorsed by the American Medical Association, AMPH soon was used to treat a plethora of medical ailments, including depression, narcolepsy, and postencephalitic Parkinson's disease (AMA Council on Pharmacy and Chemistry 1937; Cho and Segal 1994). METH and AMPH both still have an indication to treat some of these diseases (Table 2–4). Past and present military establishments have used METH and AMPH during war and peacetime operations, primarily to enhance aviation pilot concentration and reduce fatigue on long flights (Caldwell et al. 2003; Lathers and Charles 1994; Rasmussen 2009).

TABLE 2–4. Schedules and indications

Drug	Schedule	Trade name	Medical indication
Cocaine	II	Cocaine (topical)	Local anesthesia, mucous membranes; epistaxis
Amphetamine	II	Adderall, Vyvanse	ADHD, narcolepsy
Methamphetamine	II	Desoxyn	ADHD, obesity

Note. ADHD=attention-deficit/hyperactivity disorder.

Similar to AMPH, METH was first synthesized in the late 1800s by a Japanese pharmacologist (Cho and Segal 1994). METH was used during war to reduce fatigue, but it was also used by civilians working for the war effort. Around 1941, METH, like AMPH, was available over the counter in Japan as Philopon and Sedrin. The availability of METH increased dramatically after World War II (from about 1945 to 1957) because of army surpluses of the drug released onto the market. This increased availability marked the beginning of the first significant wave of METH abuse in Japan. At the same time, there was a significant increase in AMPH use in the United States after patent rights expired for the drug, allowing other companies to ramp up production (Rasmussen 2008). It has been estimated, based on conservative figures, that 5% of Japanese between the ages of 16 and 25 were either dependent on or abusing METH, but strict laws initiated in the 1950s curtailed use until the 1970s, when a second wave of METH abuse followed (Anglin et al. 2000; Cho and Segal 1994; Ujike and Sato 2004). Similar to the Japanese METH abuse estimates, one U.S. study found that during 1970–1971, 5% of American adults had used medications containing AMPH in the past year, whereas other studies obtained even higher estimates (Parry et al. 1973).

In the United States, METH quickly gained popularity in the 1960s, likely because it was inexpensive, easily manufactured in underground labs, and quickly distributed along the West Coast by motorcycle gangs (Thompson 1967). More recently, small-scale METH production (less than 2 kg per synthesis cycle) has shifted to the midwestern United States from western states (National Drug Intelligence Center 2009). These small-scale operations pale in comparison to the "superlabs" in Mexico, which are capable of producing many kilograms of METH per cycle. In fact, the latest surveillance of drug cartels indicates that Mexican superlabs have moved operations into Southern California, further challenging law enforcement on both sides of the border (National Drug Intelligence Center 2009).

Pharmacokinetics and Pharmacodynamics

The contrasting pharmacokinetics between cocaine and METH/AMPH clearly contribute to their differing behavioral and neurotoxic profiles. METH's highly addictive properties relate directly to its ability to quickly and efficiently penetrate the blood-brain barrier (Fowler et al. 2008). METH has an elimination half-life of 10–12 hours (Table 2–5). METH-dependent individuals tend to consume the drug in a binge-like pattern, though because of METH's long half-life, "binge" administration (i.e., repeated dosing over 1–3 days or more) results in accumulative concentrations of the drug that are toxic (O'Neil et al. 2006). By contrast, the half-life of cocaine is about 90 minutes, resulting in rapid clearance from the body (see Table 2–2). This relatively rapid clearance likely reduces the toxicity of cocaine relative to METH/AMPH, even though the drugs all produce acute elevations in extracellular monoamine concentrations.

METH is ingested in base and hydrochloride salt forms. A pure crystalline form of the *d* isomer is produced from the precursor ephedrine and is generally referred to as "crystal meth" because of its white appearance and assumed purity (Figure 2–11) (Beebe and Walley 1995; Cho and Melega 2002; R.B. Mack 1990). METH can be synthesized from methylamine and phenyl-2-propanone (P-2-P), though this yields a racemic mixture of the *l* and *d* isomers that is less potent than pure *d* isomer. This mixture is often tainted brown-yellow and is called "crank." A highly pure smokable form of the drug is called "ice." Following oral administration, METH is readily absorbed through the gastrointestinal tract and subsequently almost completely (90%) eliminated in urine (Caldwell 1976; Shimosato et al. 1986). At a urine pH of 6–8, most of a METH dose is excreted in urine unchanged, with 15% excreted as *p*-hydroxymethamphetamine, 4%–7% as amphetamine, and 1% as *p*-hydroxyamphetamine and other minor metabolites (Caldwell 1976; Shimosato et al. 1986). Urinary acidification increases the rate of clearance by enhancing renal excretion and thus shortening plasma elimination half-life (Beckett and Rowland 1965).

METH produces powerful sympathetic nervous system stimulation, resulting in euphoria, increased energy, and hypersexuality (Martin et al. 1971). In contrast, acute withdrawal from METH may result in transient depression, irritability, anxiety, fatigue, and hypersomnia (Newton et al. 2004). Increased sexual desire and pleasure associated with METH/AMPH consumption leads to loss of sexual inhibition and increased risk-taking behavior that appears to be more pronounced than that seen with other drugs of abuse (Frohmader et al. 2010). Of major concern is the incidence of psychosis linked to chronic METH consumption that resembles paranoid schizophrenia (Srisurapanont et al. 2003; Yui et al. 2000). Common clinical signs

TABLE 2–5. Pharmacokinetic profile of different routes of methamphetamine (METH) and amphetamine (AMPH) administration in plasma

Drug	Route of administration	Dose	N	Bio-availability	T_{max} (hours)	C_{max} (µg/L)	$t_{1/2}$ (hours)	Reference
METH	Oral[a]	10 mg	8	–	5.4	20.2	9.3	Schepers et al. 2003
		20 mg	5	–	7.5	32.4	11.1	
	IN	50 mg[b]	8	79%	2.7	37.7	10.7	Harris et al. 2003
	Oral[c]	40 mg	8	67%	2.5	41.2	10.7	
	IV	10 mg	8	–	–	–	11.4	
	Oral[d]	30 mg/kg	10	–	3.6	94.1	9.1	Shappell et al. 1996
	Oral[d]	0.125 mg/kg	6	–	3.0	22.0	–	Perez-Reyes et al. 1991
	Oral[d]	0.125 mg/kg	12	–	3.3	20.1	9.1	Cook et al. 1992
		0.250 mg/kg	12	–	2.9	39.5	11.2	
	Oral[c]	22 mg	6	–	2.5	47.1	–	Perez-Reyes et al. 1991
	Oral[c]	21.8 mg	6	90%	2.0	44.4	11.8	Cook et al. 1993
	IV	15.5 mg	6	–	4 min	101	13.1	
	Oral[e]	12.5 mg	10	–	3	20	–	Driscoll et al. 1971

TABLE 2–5. Pharmacokinetic profile of different routes of methamphetamine (METH) and amphetamine (AMPH) administration in plasma *(continued)*

Drug	Route of administration	Dose	N	Bio-availability	T_{max} (hours)	C_{max} (µg/L)	$t_{1/2}$ (hours)	Reference
AMPH	Oral[a]	10 mg	5	—	11.9	4.7	—	Schepers et al. 2003
		20 mg	5	—	14.3	5.6	—	
	IN	50 mg[b]	8	—	18.8	1.8	—	Harris et al. 2003
	Oral[c]	40 mg	8	—	16.8	2.0	—	
	Oral[c]	21.8 mg	6	—	12.0	4.2	—	Cook et al. 1993
	IV	15.5 mg	6	—	17.0	4.0	—	
	Oral[d]	0.125 mg/kg	10	—	11.7	1.6	—	Cook et al. 1992
		0.250 mg/kg	9	—	—	4.0	—	
	Oral[c]	22 mg	6	—	10–24	3–6	—	Perez-Reyes et al. 1991

Note. IN=intranasal; IV=intravenous.
[a]Desoxyn Gradumet sustained-release tablets (Abbott Laboratories).
[b]10% solution of the hydrochloride salt in an isotonic sodium chloride solution.
[c]Vapor.
[d]Capsule.
[e]Liquid solution.

of METH/AMPH-induced psychosis include auditory, visual, and tactile hallucinations and delusions (Galanter and Kleber 2008). In addition to sustained psychosis, chronic METH/AMPH dependence increases the incidence of clinically significant depression, suicidal ideation, and overdose-related mortality. Factors that may predispose an individual to develop psychosis may relate to age at onset of use, genetic susceptibility, or environmental stressors. These and other factors are topics of importance and are the focus of much needed research (Haile et al. 2009; Mahoney et al. 2010; Marshall and Werb 2010; Salo et al. 2011).

METH/AMPH administration powerfully influences central monoamine levels. While the general consensus has been that METH/AMPH's reinforcing effects are attributable more to actions on DA than to actions on other monoamines, these drugs have much more potent effects on NE (Table 2–3) (Rothman et al. 2001). However, as will be elaborated below, increases in NE may be beneficial. Indeed, NE appears to modulate METH/AMPH's effects on DAergic neurotransmission, and therefore NE could be a viable pharmacotherapeutic target for stimulant dependence (Weinshenker et al. 2002, 2008). That is, drugs that increase NE in specific brain regions may better control DA neurotransmission, whereas low NE in those brain regions would allow supraphysiological DA levels, leading to greater untoward effects. Chronic METH/AMPH consumption is associated with significant microglia-mediated inflammation and DA-induced neurotoxicity (Fleckenstein et al. 2007; Krasnova and Cadet 2009; Sulzer et al. 2005). Studies also convincingly support the idea that NE is neuroprotective and possesses anti-inflammatory effects, likely mediated by increasing *neurotrophils* and acting on astrocytes and microglia (Carnevale et al. 2007; Galea et al. 2003; Simonini et al. 2010). Blocking these neurotoxic effects may play a significant role in attenuating the pathophysiological sequelae associated with chronic METH/AMPH consumption.

Behavioral Pharmacology

As in cocaine research, animal paradigms that model human drug-taking have been important in defining METH/AMPH's reinforcing effects on behavior and neurochemistry. Preclinical and clinical behavioral pharmacology experiments conducted under highly controlled conditions show that METH and AMPH are reliably self-administered via various routes by animals and humans (Balster and Schuster 1973; Balster et al. 1976; Comer et al. 1996, 2001; De La Garza et al. 2008a; Hart et al. 2001, 2008a; Johanson et al. 1976; Newman and Carroll 2006; Newton et al. 2006; Pickens et al. 1968). METH/AMPH also serve as discriminative stimuli and substitutes for other stimulants, including cocaine (De La Garza and Johanson 1986; Li et al. 2006; Sevak et al. 2009). Depending on the dosing regimen, however, toler-

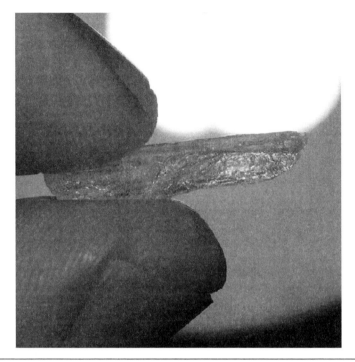

FIGURE 2–11. "Crystal meth."

A pure crystalline form of the *d* isomer of methamphetamine produced from the precursor ephedrine and generally referred to as *crystal meth* because of its white appearance and assumed purity.

Source.   See Illustration Credits at conclusion of chapter.

ance quickly develops to the positive subjective and physiological effects of METH/AMPH in humans (Brauer et al. 1996; Comer et al. 2001; C.E. Cook et al. 1993; Fischman and Schuster 1974; Perez-Reyes et al. 1991). A substantially longer period of METH/AMPH dosing is required to produce tolerance to the anorectic properties of these stimulants (Craddock 1976).

Effects on Dopamine Neurotransmission

METH has numerous mechanisms of action on central neurotransmission that relate to its reinforcing effects. Some key mechanisms to METH's effects are 1) induction of monoamine release by METH/AMPH-induced exchange diffusion, 2) reverse transport of monoamines out of neurons, 3) decreased DAT expression, and 4) decreased VMAT-2 expression (Figure 2–12). METH and AMPH are similar to cocaine in that one of their primary actions is on the DAT (Fleckenstein et al. 2007; Sulzer et al. 2005). METH/AMPH potently enhances DA levels in key limbic structures independent of neuronal depolarization (Fischer and Cho 1979). This is achieved through exchange diffusion and reverse transport processes (Fischer and Cho 1979). At high concentrations, lipophilic METH/AMPH diffuses across nerve terminal membranes and displaces intraneuronal DA, which is forced out of the cell by reverse transport (F. Mack and Bönisch 1979). Thus, METH/AMPH acts as a substrate for the DAT and competes with DA at the substrate-binding site that inhibits DAT function. By contrast, cocaine inhibits the DAT but without causing monoamine release at a different site that still appears to interact with METH/AMPH's site (Wayment et al. 1998). This interaction may relate to why formulated AMPH and METH have proved efficacious for cocaine dependence as described in anecdotal case reports and demonstrated in a number of clinical trials (Grabowski et al. 2001, 2004; Haile et al. 2010; Herin et al. 2010; Mooney et al. 2009). Other drugs that act at the DAT and NET, such as bupropion and methylphenidate, have also shown promise for METH/AMPH dependence (Elkashef et al. 2008; Newton et al. 2005b, 2006; Rau et al. 2005; Shoptaw et al. 2008; Tiihonen et al. 2007).

METH and AMPH significantly usurp normal neurophysiology in brain reward areas that contribute to their potent reinforcing effects related to DA neurotransmission. For example, METH enhances mesolimbic VTA cell body neuron responses to subsequent administrations of METH, an effect that is Ca^{2+} channel– and D_2 receptor–dependent (Amano et al. 2003; Uramura et al. 2000). In vitro intracellular recordings in brain slices of animals previously administered METH also show postsynaptic sensitization of D_1 receptor–mediated hyperpolarizations in the NAc (Higashi et al. 1989). Pretreatment with DA antagonists does indeed attenuate some of METH's effects on neurophysiology and some of its behavioral effects in animals (Ujike et al. 1989; Witkin et al. 1999). However, treatment with the nonselective DA antagonist haloperidol or the more selective D_2 antagonist risperidone does not block all the positive subjective effects of METH in humans (Wachtel and de Wit 1999).

It has been difficult to apply preclinical findings in animal models to the human clinical arena because of the lack of evidence of persistent brain changes. While changes in DAT and DA receptor subtypes are seen at acute withdrawal in animals that have been self-administering METH, these alterations do not persist (Stefanski et al. 1999, 2002). Animals with long-term histories of self-administering METH do have decreased DAT protein levels in the PFC and ventral striatum that persist after withdrawal but not in other areas implicated in mediating drug reinforcement (Schwendt et al. 2009).

In contrast, structural and neurophysiological neuroadaptations do appear to endure and may apply to humans, though clinical research understandably lags behind preclinical research in this area. Studies show that METH/AMPH alters dendritic complexity and spine density in medium

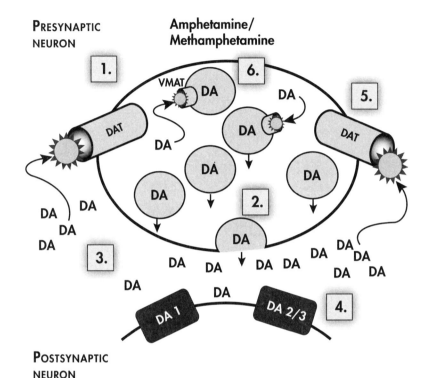

1. DA neuron activation
2. Potently induces vesicular DA mobilization to terminals and release
3. AMPH/METH increases neurotransmitter in the synaptic cleft
4. Monoamine receptor subtypes activated
5. AMPH/METH prevents the inactivation of DA by altering the DAT
6. AMPH/METH prevents repackaging of DA by altering the VMAT

FIGURE 2–12. Mechanisms of action on central neurotransmission that relate to the reinforcing effects of methamphetamine (METH) and amphetamine (AMPH).

DA=dopamine; DAT=dopamine transporter; VMAT=vesicular monoamine transporter.

spiny neurons in the NAc VTA DAergic neurons, and PFC pyramidal neurons (Robinson and Kolb 1997, 2004; Russo et al. 2010). Altered complexity and spine density relate to LTD and LTP, cellular forms of synaptic plasticity implicated in learning and memory and other processes (Bourne and Harris 2007). As mentioned previously, LTD is associated with spine retraction and shrinkage. In contrast, LTP is associated with the generation of new and bigger spines (Matsuzaki et al. 2004; Nägerl et al. 2004; Okamoto et al. 2004).

These persistent changes in morphology are linked to the expression of AMPA GLU receptors that have been implicated in the reinforcing effects of stimulants in animals (Carlezon and Nestler 2002; Holtmaat et al. 2005). As seen with cocaine treatment, METH/AMPH-induced synaptic plasticity involves altering LTP and mobilizing cytoskeletal proteins, CREB, CDK5, and structure-specific alterations of BDNF levels that affect DA neurotransmission (Angelucci et al. 2007; P. Chen and Chen 2005; Narita et al. 2003; Skelton et al. 2007; Swant et al. 2010). More research is needed on the possibility of preventing drug-induced neuroplasticity and whether this offers any therapeutic advantage as it relates to METH/AMPH dependence.

Mechanisms of Neurotoxicity

The mechanisms responsible for METH/AMPH-induced toxicity have been extensively researched, and the reader is urged to refer to many excellent reviews on this topic (Fleckenstein et al. 2007; Krasnova and Cadet 2009; Reiner et al. 2009; Sulzer et al. 2005; Yamamoto et al. 2010). Briefly, some key mechanisms are oxidative stress linked to DA, excitotoxicity, hyperthermia, and neuroinflammation.

Oxidative stress linked to DA. METH/AMPH administration redistributes cytosolic DA for immediate release by inactivating the vesicular monoamine transporter–2 (VMAT-2) that is responsible for neurotransmitter repackaging and storage (Eyerman and Yamamoto 2007; Liu and Edwards 1997; Riddle et al. 2002). It inactivates VMAT-2 by producing supraphysiological levels of synaptic DA that are auto-oxidized into highly reactive species, *decreasing* DAT and VMAT-2 and further *increasing* neurotoxic intraneuronal DA (Figure 2–12) (Berman et al. 1996; Fleckenstein et al. 1997). DA receptor antagonists such as eticlopride, DAT blockers, and DA depletion attenuate METH's effects on the DAT and prevent decreases in VMAT-2 (Brown et al. 2002; Metzger et al. 2000).

Similarly, DA metabolized by the enzyme monoamine oxidase increases levels of hydrogen peroxide that interacts with metal ions forming toxic hydroxyl radicals deadly to neurons (Melega et al. 2007). Drugs that block DA synthesis and DA receptors attenuate METH/AMPH-induced toxicity, whereas those that promote DA production exacerbate these effects (O'Dell et al. 1993; D.M. Thomas et al. 2008). Moreover, pretreatment with antioxidants protects neurons from damage, which is consistent with oxidative stress–mediated toxicity attributed to METH/AMPH administration (Fukami et al. 2004; Hashimoto et al. 2004).

Excitotoxicity. Another well-researched line of evidence implicated in the neurotoxicity of METH/AMPH suggests that GLUergic excitotoxic mechanisms are involved. Mechanisms acting primarily through the NMDA receptor GLU subtype in tandem with DA appear to play a significant role in METH/AMPH-associated toxic effects in brain (Sonsalla et al. 1989). For example, NMDA antagonists block some of the toxic effects of METH/AMPH treatment on nigrostriatal neurons (Sonsalla et al. 1991). METH/AMPH-sustained increases in GLU and subsequent overstimulation of NMDA receptors have been linked to formation of superoxide radicals, nitric oxide (NO), and neural toxicity (Sheng et al. 1996). NO reacts with superoxide radicals to form the potent neurotoxin peroxynitrite (Pacher et al. 2007). Neurotoxicity attributed to peroxynitrite metabolites and DA depletion is attenuated by selective NO inhibitors and potent antioxidants (Eyerman and Yamamoto 2007; Imam and Ali 2000; Imam et al. 1999).

Hyperthermia.   Studies also demonstrate that the potent hyperthermic effects of METH enhance production of reactive oxygen species that further contribute to its neurotoxic effects by increasing the formation of DA quinones, which adversely affects the DAT, injures DA neurons, and increases free radical levels (Kil et al. 1996; LaVoie and Hastings 1999; Numachi et al. 2007; Whitehead et al. 2001; Xie et al. 2000). In contrast, blocking NMDA receptors or neutralizing METH's hyperthermic properties attenuates some of these pathological characteristics (Ali et al. 1996; Bowyer et al. 2001; Miller and O'Callaghan 1994). Hyperthermia associated with METH/AMPH administration also compromises the blood-brain barrier, which further potentiates damage to neurons and glial, vascular endothelium, and myelin destruction (Kiyatkin and Sharma 2009a, 2009b; Ramirez et al. 2009).

Neuroinflammation.   Some research indicates that microglial activation and subsequent inflammatory processes contribute to neurodegeneration and cell death. Indeed, METH's microglial activation is swift, resulting in significant neural damage that is blocked by NMDA antagonists and anti-inflammatory agents (Asanuma et al. 2003; Sriram et al. 2006; D.M. Thomas et al. 2004, 2008; L. Zhang et al. 2006). Whether medications that block NMDA receptors or anti-inflammatory agents may prove effective for METH/AMPH-dependent individuals is unknown. Further research addressing these questions is needed.

Norepinephrine Neurotransmission

Recent evidence has brought NE back to the research forefront, highlighting its importance in different aspects of stimulant dependence (Sofuoglu and Sewell 2009; Weinshenker and Schroeder 2007). Indeed, various lines of research suggest that NE modulates DA, since depletion of NE significantly enhances METH's ability to increase and subsequently deplete DA (Fornai et al.

1998; Preseton et al. 1985). Similarly, administration of the dopamine β-hydroxylase (DβH) inhibitor fusaric acid, which prevents the synthesis of NE, and genetic ablation of the DβH gene in mice both increase the neurotoxic and behavioral effects of METH (Weinshenker et al. 2008). DβH-deficient mice are also hypersensitive to the behavioral effects of AMPH (Weinshenker et al. 2002). Drugs that bind to different adrenergic receptors have helped reveal which specific subtype may be mediating METH/AMPH effects. For example, treatment with clonidine, a drug that shuts off NE release by stimulating presynaptic α_2-adrenergic autoreceptors, potentiates METH-induced effects, whereas blockade of α_2-adrenergic receptors with antagonists (yohimbine) is protective (Fornai et al. 1998). Likewise, blocking α_1-adrenergic receptors with prazosin in the NAc decreases endogenous DA release, and when infused in the PFC, prazosin decreases AMPH-induced locomotor activation (Darracq et al. 1998). METH's behavioral effects and AMPH-induced increases in DA are also attenuated in genetically altered mice lacking the α_1-adrenergic receptor subtype (Auclair et al. 2002; Battaglia et al. 2003). These studies highlight the α_1-adrenergic receptor subtype as a promising therapeutic target for treating neurotoxicity and the potent reinforcing effects related to METH/AMPH dependence in humans. Medications that block α_1-adrenergic receptors are used clinically in humans as antihypertensives.

Results from human studies are consistent with the notion that NE may modulate the subjective effects of METH/AMPH. For example, 4 days of disulfiram (250 mg), which blocks the production of NE, *enhances* many of AMPH's (20 mg/70 kg) positive and negative subjective effects (Sofuoglu et al. 2008). In contrast, increasing NEergic neurotransmission with the NET reuptake inhibitor atomoxetine attenuates some of the subjective and cardiovascular effects of AMPH (Sofuoglu et al. 2009). Other drugs that act on the NEergic system have shown promise in preclinical models of relapse to METH self-administration. The wake-promoting drug modafinil, which blocks the DAT and NET (leading to increased NE neurotransmission), blocks context-induced, cue-induced, and drug-primed reinstatement to METH self-administration (Mitchell and Weinshenker 2010; Reichel and See 2010). Mirtazapine, a medication that also blocks α_2-adrenergic receptors, was recently shown to attenuate cue-induced METH reinstatement to drug taking (Graves and Napier 2011). Clinical studies in METH-dependent individuals show positive effects of mirtazapine treatment on withdrawal symptoms associated with detoxification (Cruickshank et al. 2008; Kongsakon et al. 2005; McGregor et al. 2008). Although larger clinical trials are needed, small pilot studies continue to support both mirtazapine and modafinil as promising pharmacotherapy for METH dependence (McElhiney et al. 2009; Shearer et al. 2009).

Glutamate Neurotransmission

METH/AMPH potently alters GLU, the most abundant excitatory neuro-transmitter in the brain. GLU neurotransmission and levels are largely maintained by glial release and transport (Hassel et al. 2003; Ziskin et al. 2007). Glial cells also express different GLU receptor subtypes (Káradóttir et al. 2005). Although mostly thought to contribute to the neurotoxic effects of METH, GLU in the PFC plays a central role in mediating psychostimulant reinstatement of self-administration in animals, although other brain areas are involved (Figure 2–3) (Kalivas 2009; Knackstedt and Kalivas 2009; Sulzer et al. 2005; Yahyavi-Firouz-Abadi and See 2009). This idea applied in humans to METH/AMPH-dependent individuals would suggest that drug-induced impairments in levels of GLU in the PFC (and GLU projections to areas such as the NAc) render individuals vulnerable to relapse after a period of abstinence (Danbolt 2001; Gorelova and Yang 1997; Kalivas 2009; Knackstedt and Kalivas 2009). Consistent with this line of evidence, rodent studies demonstrate that PFC GLU released into the NAc is essential for reinstatement of psychostimulant self-administration and that levels are persistently compromised after drug exposure (McFarland et al. 2003; Moussawi et al. 2011). Moreover, human imaging studies in METH-dependent individuals clearly indicate disrupted GLU neurotransmission and glial compromise that are also localized primarily to the PFC (Ernst and Chang 2008; Sailasuta et al. 2010a, 2010b).

How GLU may mediate METH's potent reinforcing effects is unknown. Evidence from mice lacking a specific metabotropic GLU receptor (mGluR5) that appear to be unresponsive to the behavioral activating and reinforcing effects of cocaine suggests this receptor subtype may be important for METH's action (Chiamulera et al. 2001). Consistent with the effects on cocaine, compounds that block mGluR5 receptors also attenuate the reinforcing effects of drug-induced reinstatement of METH self-administration (Gass et al. 2009). PFC GLU regulates DAergic neurons in the NAc, and mGluR5 antagonists block METH-induced increases in DA in this area, suggesting that this receptor may be an important therapeutic target (Tokunaga et al. 2009). Clinical testing of medications targeting the mGluR5 receptor for METH dependence in humans is warranted.

Although much evidence supports GLU's role in METH/AMPH effects, few studies have been conducted, mainly because of a lack of medications that specifically target GLU. As noted previously, N-acetylcysteine is a medication that is metabolized into cysteine and cystine (cystine consists of two cysteine molecules), which are transported into cells by cystine-glutamate exchange, whereby intracellular GLU is exchanged with cystine, thus increasing interneuronal GLU (McBean 2002). A number of studies show that

N-acetylcysteine reverses cocaine's behavioral and biochemical effects (see subsection "Effects on Glutamate Neurotransmission" earlier in this chapter), and evidence suggests similar attenuation of METH/AMPH's effects (Achat-Mendes et al. 2007; Fukami et al. 2004; Hashimoto et al. 2004; X. Zhang et al. 2009).

The antibiotic minocycline, used to treat acne, also alters central GLU, attenuates AMPH-induced DA release and behavioral activation, and blocks METH's deleterious effects on the DAT and microglial activation linked to inflammation (Hashimoto et al. 2007; Imbesi et al. 2008; Suzuki et al. 2010; L. Zhang et al. 2006, 2007). Further, minocycline treatment was shown to significantly attenuate some of the subjective effects of experimentally delivered AMPH in humans (Sofuoglu et al. 2011). There was a recent case report of a METH-dependent patient with psychotic features who was successfully treated with minocycline when antipsychotic treatment failed (Tanibuchi et al. 2010).

Although modafinil's primary action is on the DAT and NET, this medication also increases central GLU levels (Ferraro et al. 1997). Results from clinical studies assessing modafinil as a possible treatment for METH/AMPH dependence remain promising (De La Garza et al. 2010; Heinzerling et al. 2010; Kalechstein et al. 2010; McElhiney et al. 2009; McGaugh et al. 2009; Shearer et al. 2009). Taken together, evidence continues to accumulate that GLU plays an important role in the development of pharmacotherapies for METH/AMPH dependence. The future availability of pharmacologically specific ligands to GLU receptors will greatly enhance this process.

Neural Deficiencies in METH/AMPH Dependence: Pharmacotherapeutic Targets

Neuroimaging studies have consistently demonstrated that METH use, by any route, can cause profound adverse changes in brain chemistry, morphology, and neurotransmission that adversely affect overall function and neurocognition (Scott et al. 2007). Indeed, METH/AMPH-dependent individuals have significant abnormalities in global brain function (Kalechstein et al. 2009; Newton et al. 2003; Volkow et al. 2001b). As mentioned, METH/AMPH-dependent individuals have decreased DAT binding in the PFC and other important brain areas linked to relapse as measured with positron emission tomography (PET) imaging (McCann et al. 1998). Decreased DAT binding in these areas has been observed in recently detoxified individuals and in those who have been abstinent for nearly a year (Iyo et al. 2004; Sekine et al. 2001; Volkow et al. 2001b). METH-induced psychosis and psychomotor impairment are correlated with decreased striatal DAT levels (Sekine et al. 2001; Volkow et al. 2001a). Medications that either block METH's effects on the DAT or correct DAT deficiencies may mitigate some of the psychiatric sequelae associated with METH dependence.

METH/AMPH dependence is associated with significant neurocognitive deficits (Kalechstein et al. 2003). More specifically, METH dependence is accompanied by impairments in memory recall, working memory, impulsivity, attention, perseveration, and fluency (Kalechstein et al. 2003; Scott et al. 2007). Recent work has focused on reversing cognitive impairment as a strategy for therapeutic intervention for stimulant dependence (Sofuoglu 2010). Consistent with this theory, medications that enhance cognition by increasing DA, NE, GLU, or ACh levels appear promising for METH/AMPH dependence. For example, increasing ACh levels by blocking the enzymes acetylcholinesterase and/or butyrylcholinesterase, which break down ACh, with rivastigmine blocks some of the subjective and cardiovascular effects of METH in humans (De La Garza et al. 2008a, 2008b). The NET inhibitor and ADHD medication atomoxetine improves response inhibition and impulsivity that are compromised in METH/AMPH-dependent individuals. Further, atomoxetine also blocks some of the positive subjective and cardiovascular effects of AMPH in humans (Chamberlain et al. 2007; Sofuoglu et al. 2009). Similar effects have been achieved with modafinil (De La Garza et al. 2010; Turner et al. 2004). Future large-scale studies directly assessing these and other cognitive enhancers for METH/AMPH dependence are needed.

Decreased D_2 receptors appear to be a common abnormality in drug-dependent individuals across drug classes and another viable therapeutic target for METH/AMPH dependence. For instance, alcoholic individuals and opioid-, cocaine-, and METH-dependent individuals all have significantly reduced D_2 receptor levels (Fowler et al. 2001; Martinez et al. 2004; Volkow et al. 1990, 1996a; Wang et al. 1997). Low expression of D_2 receptors in drug-dependent individuals is associated with altered drug-induced euphoria and drug craving (Volkow et al. 1996b, 1999b). Similarly, PET imaging in drug-naïve rats indicates that low levels of D_2 receptors in the ventral striatum (an area that includes the NAc) predict impulsivity and greater stimulant self-administration (Dalley et al. 2007). Rodents that have a greater propensity to self-administer drugs of abuse across drug classes also have low D_2 receptors and, correspondingly, altered responses to DAergic agents (Flores et al. 1998; Haile and Kosten 2001; Maldonado et al. 1997; Stefanini et al. 1992). Likewise, genetic ablation of the D_2 receptor in mice significantly decreases the rewarding effects of stimulants (Haile et al. 2007). These data suggest an important role for D_2 receptors in METH/AMPH dependence and underscore them as a possible therapeutic target. Indeed, the ADHD medication methylphenidate and antidepressant medication bupropion both increase D_2 receptor levels and have been shown to either attenuate METH/AMPH's subjective effects or decrease METH/AMPH use in METH/AMPH-dependent individuals (Elkashef et al. 2008; Newton et al. 2005b, 2006; Shoptaw et al. 2008; Thanos et al. 2007; Tiihonen et al. 2007; Vassout et al. 1993).

Conclusion

Preclinical and clinical studies continue to define the complex pharmacology and pharmacodynamics of the action of cocaine and METH/AMPH from the molecular to the behavioral level. Different forms of these drugs differ in their addictive potency, which is related to how quickly the drug traverses the blood-brain barrier and affects key limbic circuits. Research determining cocaine's and METH/AMPH's ability to induce aberrant synaptic plasticity on brain circuits linked to reward learning is especially insightful. Human imaging studies have identified deficiencies in limbic brain areas related to DA neurotransmission that may perhaps signal a vulnerable phenotype prone to develop psychostimulant dependence. These insights further support psychostimulant dependence as a brain disease in need of appropriate, efficacious treatment. Clinical studies to date have switched focus from the DAergic to the NEergic and GLUergic neurotransmitter systems and have given rise to promising pharmacotherapies and new avenues of inquiry.

KEY CLINICAL CONCEPTS

- The coca plant (*Erythroxylon coca*) has been used for thousands of years for its medicinal properties. Although presently used medicinally, extracted pure cocaine is a highly addictive psychostimulant that is used in different forms and ingested or administered through various routes.

- Cocaine blocks dopamine (DA), norepinephrine (NE), and serotonin reuptake, increasing synaptic levels of these neurotransmitters to supraphysiological levels. Cocaine also disrupts central basal glutamate (GLU) levels. Changes in neurotransmitter levels within the mesocorticolimbic system correlate with cocaine's euphoric effects and drug craving.

- The reinforcing effects of cocaine are generally linked to DA. However, accumulating evidence indicates NE and GLU appear to play an even more important role in cocaine's positive subjective effects and in relapse to drug taking.

- Numerous molecular mechanisms are altered by cocaine administration, and many play key roles in mediating neural plasticity associated with learning processes. Cocaine-induced neural plasticity within vital reinforcement-related brain circuitry may be long-lasting and linked to continued relapse after a period of abstinence.

- Cocaine-dependent individuals have decreased DA synthesis, reduced endogenous DA levels, blunted stimulant-induced DA release, reduced D_2/D_3 receptor availability, and increased dopamine transporter (DAT) and cortical NE transporter levels.

- A substantial number of clinical trials have identified compounds that theoretically may correct deficiencies in neural circuits and attenuate the reinforcing effects of cocaine in cocaine-dependent individuals. Some also appear to block drug cue–induced craving that relates to relapse. These compounds include DA releasers such as medications used to treat attention-deficit/hyperactivity disorder in sustained-release formulations that have low abuse liability; mixed DA reuptake inhibitors (modafinil); DA precursors (L-dopa); NE synthesis blockers (disulfiram); and drugs that potentiate GLU neurotransmission (*N*-acetylcysteine).

- METH and AMPH have a long history of illicit and therapeutic use the world over.

- METH's and AMPH's contrasting pharmacokinetics compared with cocaine contribute toward their powerful behavioral and neurotoxic profiles.

- METH and AMPH have profound effects on brain DA, NE, and GLU neurotransmission that mediate these drugs' reinforcing effects and contribute toward deficits in overall neurocognitive functioning.

- Chronic METH/AMPH use is linked to aberrant synaptic plasticity and decreased DAT, D_2 receptors, and vesicular monoamine transporter–2, as well as to substantial neurotoxicity. Some prominent mechanisms associated with METH/AMPH-induced neurotoxicity include DA-mediated oxidative stress, excitotoxicity, hyperthermia, and neuroinflammation.

- Cognitive enhancers and anti-inflammatory agents have shown promise for METH/AMPH dependence. This suggests that perhaps a combination of anti-addictive and neuroprotective medications may be needed to help address multisystem deficits associated with this dependency.

Resources

Cocaine

Journal Articles

Berridge KC, Robinson TE, Aldridge JW: Dissecting components of reward: "liking," "wanting," and learning. Curr Opin Pharmacol 9:65–73, 2009

Everitt BJ, Robbins TW: Neural systems of reinforcement for drug addiction: from actions to habits to compulsion. Nat Neurosci 8:1481–1489, 2005

Herin DV, Rush CR, Grabowski J: Agonist-like pharmacotherapy for stimulant dependence: preclinical, human laboratory, and clinical studies. Ann N Y Acad Sci 1187:76–100, 2010

Kalivas PW: The glutamate homeostasis hypothesis of addiction. Nat Rev Neurosci 10:561–572, 2009

Koob GF, Volkow ND: Neurocircuitry of addiction. Neuropsychopharmacology 35:217–238, 2010

Nutt D, King LA, Saulsbury W, et al: Development of a rational scale to assess the harm of drugs of potential misuse. Lancet 369:1047–1053, 2007

Russo SJ, Dietz DM, Dumitriu D, et al: The addicted synapse: mechanisms of synaptic and structural plasticity in nucleus accumbens. Trends Neurosci 33:267–276, 2010

Weinshenker D, Schroeder JP: There and back again: a tale of norepinephrine and drug addiction. Neuropsychopharmacology 32:1433–1451, 2007

Books

Ries RK, Fiellin DA, Miller SC, et al (eds): Principles of Addiction Medicine, 4th Edition. Philadephia, PA, Lippincott Williams & Wilkins, 2009

Websites

National Institutes of Health
http://drugabuse.gov/nidahome.html

U.S. National Library of Medicine
http://druginfo.nlm.nih.gov/drugportal/drugportal.jsp

Frequently asked questions about cocaine for the general inquirer
http://www.thegooddrugsguide.com/cocaine/faq.htm

Methamphetamine and Amphetamine

Journal Articles

Fleckenstein AE, Volz TJ, Riddle EL, et al: New insights into the mechanism of action of amphetamines. Annu Rev Pharmacol Toxicol 47:681–698, 2007

Fowler JS, Volkow ND, Logan J, et al: Fast uptake and long-lasting binding of methamphetamine in the human brain: comparison with cocaine. Neuroimage 43:756–763, 2008

Karila L, Weinstein A, Aubin HJ, et al: Pharmacological approaches to methamphetamine dependence: a focused review. Br J Clin Pharmacol 69:578–592, 2010

Krasnova IN, Cadet JL: Methamphetamine toxicity and messengers of death. Brain Res Rev 60:379–407, 2009

Rasmussen N: America's first amphetamine epidemic 1929–1971: a quantitative and qualitative retrospective with implications for the present. Am J Public Health 98:974–985, 2008

Sulzer D, Sonders MS, Poulsen NW, et al: Mechanisms of neurotransmitter release by amphetamines: a review. Prog Neurobiol 75:406–433, 2005

Volkow ND, Wang GJ, Fowler JS, et al: Addiction: decreased reward sensitivity and increased expectation sensitivity conspire to overwhelm the brain's control circuit. Bioessays 32:748–755, 2010

Books

Rasmussen N: On Speed: The Many Lives of Amphetamine. New York, New York University Press, 2009

Websites

Comprehensive index on METH-related literature from a number of sources
http://www.nyhealth.gov/diseases/aids/harm_reduction/crystalmeth/docs/ meth_literature_index.pdf

U.S. National Library of Medicine
http://druginfo.nlm.nih.gov/drugportal/drugportal.jsp

Internet videos related to METH/AMPH
http://www.abc.net.au/4corners/special_eds/20060320/
http://www.pbs.org/wgbh/pages/frontline/meth/

Frequently asked questions about METH/AMPH for the general inquirer
http://www.thegooddrugsguide.com/amphetamines/faq.htm

References

Achat-Mendes C, Anderson KL, Itzhak Y: Impairment in consolidation of learned place preference following dopaminergic neurotoxicity in mice is ameliorated by N-acetylcysteine but not D1 and D2 dopamine receptor agonists. Neuropsychopharmacology 32:531–541, 2007

Adewale AS, Platt DM, Spealman RD: Pharmacological stimulation of group ii me-
    tabotropic glutamate receptors reduces cocaine self-administration and cocaine-
    induced reinstatement of drug seeking in squirrel monkeys. J Psychopharmacol
    Exp Ther 318:922–931, 2006
Ahmed SH, Koob GF: Cocaine- but not food-seeking behavior is reinstated by stress
    after extinction. Psychopharmacology 132:289–295, 1997
Alhassoon OM, Dupont RM, Schweinsburg BC, et al: Regional cerebral blood flow in
    cocaine- versus methamphetamine-dependent patients with a history of alco-
    holism. Int J Neuropsychopharmacol 4:105–112, 2001
Ali SF, Newport GD, Slikker W: Methamphetamine-induced dopaminergic toxicity in
    mice. Role of environmental temperature and pharmacological agents. Ann N Y
    Acad Sci 801:187–198, 1996
Alles G: The comparative physiological actions of dl-β-phenylisopropylamines, I:
    pressor effect and toxicity. J Pharmacol Exp Ther 47:339–354, 1933
AMA Council on Pharmacy and Chemistry: Present status of Benzedrine sulfate.
    JAMA 109:2064–2069, 1937
Amano T, Matsubayashi H, Seki T, et al: Repeated administration of methamphet-
    amine causes hypersensitivity of D2 receptor in rat ventral tegmental area. Neu-
    rosci Lett 347:89–92, 2003
Anderson AL, Reid MS, Li SH, et al: Modafinil for the treatment of cocaine depen-
    dence. Drug Alcohol Depend 104:133–139, 2009
Ang E, Chen J, Zagouras P, et al: Induction of nuclear factor-kappaB in nucleus ac-
    cumbens by chronic cocaine administration. J Neurochem 79:221–224, 2001
Angarita GA, Pittman B, Gueorguieva R, et al: Regulation of cocaine self-administra-
    tion in humans: lack of evidence for loading and maintenance phases. Pharma-
    col Biochem Behav 95:51–55, 2010
Angelucci F, Gruber SH, El Khoury A, et al: Chronic amphetamine treatment reduces
    NGF and BDNF in the rat brain. Eur Neuropsychopharmacol 17:756–762, 2007
Anglin MD, Burke C, Perrochet B, et al: History of the methamphetamine problem.
    J Psychoactive Drugs 32:137–141, 2000
Anwyl R: Metabotropic glutamate receptors: electrophysiological properties and role
    in plasticity. Brain Res Brain Res Rev 29:83–120, 1999
Argilli E, Sibley DR, Malenka RC, et al: Mechanism and time course of cocaine-
    induced long-term potentiation in the ventral tegmental area. J Neurosci
    28(37):9092–9100, 2008. doi:10.1523/JNEUROSCI.1001-08.2008
Asanuma M, Tsuji T, Miyazaki I, et al: Methamphetamine-induced neurotoxicity in
    mouse brain is attenuated by ketoprofen, a non-steroidal anti-inflammatory
    drug. Neurosci Lett 352:13–16, 2003
Auclair A, Cotecchia S, Glowinski J, et al: D-Amphetamine fails to increase extracel-
    lular dopamine levels in mice lacking alpha 1b-adrenergic receptors: relation-
    ship between functional and nonfunctional dopamine release. J Neurosci
    22:9150–9154, 2002
Bäckström P, Hyytiä P: Ionotropic and metabotropic glutamate receptor antagonism
    attenuates cue-induced cocaine seeking. Neuropsychopharmacology 31:778–
    786, 2006
Bäckström P, Hyytiä P: Involvement of AMPA/kainate, NMDA, and mGlu5 receptors
    in the nucleus accumbens core in cue-induced reinstatement of cocaine seeking
    in rats. Psychopharmacology (Berl) 192:571–580, 2007

Baker DA, Shen H, Kalivas PW: Cystine/glutamate exchange serves as the source for extracellular glutamate: modifications by repeated cocaine administration. Amino Acids 23:161–162, 2002

Baker DA, McFarland K, Lake RW, et al: Neuroadaptations in cystine-glutamate exchange underlie cocaine relapse. Nat Neurosci 6:743–749, 2003

Baker JR, Jatlow P, McCance-Katz EF: Disulfiram effects on responses to intravenous cocaine administration. Drug Alcohol Depend 87:202–209, 2007

Balleine BW, Dickinson A: Goal-directed instrumental action: contingency and incentive learning and their cortical substrates. Neuropharmacology 37:407–419, 1998

Balster RL, Schuster CR: A comparison of d-amphetamine, l-amphetamine, and methamphetamine self-administration in rhesus monkeys. Pharmacol Biochem Behav 1:67–71, 1973

Balster RL, Kilbey MM, Ellinwood EH: Methamphetamine self-administration in the cat. Psychopharmacologia 46:229–233, 1976

Barr GA, Sharpless NS, Cooper S, et al: Classical conditioning, decay and extinction of cocaine-induced hyperactivity and stereotypy. Life Sci 33:1341–1351, 1983

Battaglia G, Fornai F, Busceti CL, et al: Alpha-1B adrenergic receptor knockout mice are protected against methamphetamine toxicity. J Neurochem 86:413–421, 2003

Beckett AH, Rowland M: Urinary excretion of methylamphetamine in man. Nature 206:1260–1261, 1965

Beebe DK, Walley E: Smokable methamphetamine ("ice"): an old drug in a different form. Am Fam Physician 51:449–453, 1995

Berman SB, Zigmond MJ, Hastings TG: Modification of dopamine transporter function: effect of reactive oxygen species and dopamine. J Neurochem 67:593–600, 1996

Berridge KC, Robinson TE, Aldridge JW: Dissecting components of reward: "liking," "wanting," and learning. Curr Opin Pharmacol 9:65–73, 2009

Bindra D: A motivational view of learning, performance, and behavior modification. Psychol Rev 81:199–213, 1974

Blanc G, Trovero F, Vezina P, et al: Blockade of prefronto-cortical alpha 1-adrenergic receptors prevents locomotor hyperactivity induced by subcortical D-amphetamine injection. Eur J Neurosci 6:293–298, 1994

Bourne J, Harris KM: Do thin spines learn to be mushroom spines that remember? Curr Opin Neurobiol 17:381–386, 2007

Bowers MS, Chen BT, Bonci A: AMPA receptor synaptic plasticity induced by psychostimulants: the past, present, and therapeutic future. Neuron 67:11–24, 2010

Bowyer JF, Holson RR, Miller DB, et al: Phenobarbital and dizocilpine can block methamphetamine-induced neurotoxicity in mice by mechanisms that are independent of thermoregulation. Brain Res 919:179–183, 2001

Brauer LH, Ambre J, De Wit H: Acute tolerance to subjective but not cardiovascular effects of d-amphetamine in normal, healthy men. J Clin Psychopharmacol 16:72–76, 1996

Broadbent J, Gaspard TM, Dworkin SI: Assessment of the discriminative stimulus effects of cocaine in the rat: lack of interaction with opioids. Pharmacol Biochem Behav 51:379–385, 1995

Brown JM, Riddle EL, Sandoval V, et al: A single methamphetamine administration rapidly decreases vesicular dopamine uptake. J Pharmacol Exp Ther 302:497–501, 2002

Brunt TM, Rigter S, Hoek J, et al: An analysis of cocaine powder in the Netherlands: content and health hazards due to adulterants. Addiction 104:798–805, 2009

Caine SB, Koob GF: Modulation of cocaine self-administration in the rat through D-3 dopamine receptors. Science 260:1814–1816, 1993

Caldwell J: The metabolism of amphetamines in mammals. Drug Metab Rev 5:219–280, 1976

Caldwell JA, Caldwell JL, Darlington KK: Utility of dextroamphetamine for attenuating the impact of sleep deprivation in pilots. Aviat Space Environ Med 74:1125–1134, 2003

Carlezon WA, Nestler EJ: Elevated levels of GluR1 in the midbrain: a trigger for sensitization to drugs of abuse? Trends Neurosci 25:610–615, 2002

Carlezon WA, Duman RS, Nestler EJ: The many faces of CREB. Trends Neurosci 28:436–445, 2005

Carlisle HJ, Kennedy MB: Spine architecture and synaptic plasticity. Trends Neurosci 28:182–187, 2005

Carnevale D, De Simone R, Minghetti L: Microglia-neuron interaction in inflammatory and degenerative diseases: role of cholinergic and noradrenergic systems. CNS Neurol Disord Drug Targets 6:388–397, 2007

Carroll KM, Nich C, Ball SA, et al: Treatment of cocaine and alcohol dependence with psychotherapy and disulfiram. Addiction 93:713–727, 1998

Carroll KM, Fenton LR, Ball SA, et al: Efficacy of disulfiram and cognitive behavior therapy in cocaine-dependent outpatients: a randomized placebo-controlled trial. Arch Gen Psychiatry 61:264–272, 2004

Castells X, Casas M, Pérez-Mañá C, et al: Efficacy of psychostimulant drugs for cocaine dependence. Cochrane Database of Systematic Reviews 2010, Issue 2. Art. No.: CD007380. DOI: 10.1002/14651858. CD007380.pub3.

Centers for Disease Control and Prevention: Agranulocytosis associated with cocaine use—four states, March 2008–November 2009. MMWR Morb Mortal Wkly Rep 58:1381–1385, 2009

Chamberlain SR, Del Campo N, Dowson J, et al: Atomoxetine improved response inhibition in adults with attention deficit/hyperactivity disorder. Biol Psychiatry 62:977–984, 2007

Chen BT, Bowers MS, Martin M, et al: Cocaine but not natural reward self-administration nor passive cocaine infusion produces persistent LTP in the VTA. Neuron 59:288–297, 2008

Chen P, Chen J: Enhanced Cdk5 activity and p35 translocation in the ventral striatum of acute and chronic methamphetamine-treated rats. Neuropsychopharmacology 30:538–549, 2005

Chiamulera C, Epping-Jordan MP, Zocchi A, et al: Reinforcing and locomotor stimulant effects of cocaine are absent in mGluR5 null mutant mice. Nat Neurosci 4:873–874, 2001

Chiodo KA, Läck CM, Roberts DCS: Cocaine self-administration reinforced on a progressive ratio schedule decreases with continuous D-amphetamine treatment in rats. Psychopharmacology (Berl) 200:465–473, 2008

Cho AK, Melega WP: Patterns of methamphetamine abuse and their consequences. J Addict Dis 21:21–34, 2002

Cho AK, Segal DS: Amphetamine and Its Analogs: Psychopharmacology, Toxicology, and Abuse, 1st Edition. New York, Academic Press, 1994

Clement B, Goff C, Forbes TDA: Toxic amines and alkaloids from *Acacia berlandieri.* Phytochemistry 46:249–254, 1997

Clement B, Goff C, Forbes TDA: Toxic amines and alkaloids from *Acacia rigidula.* Phytochemistry 49:1377–1380, 1998

Collins RJ, Weeks JR, Cooper MM, et al: Prediction of abuse liability of drugs using IV self-administration by rats. Psychopharmacology 82:6–13, 1984

Colpaert FC, Niemegeers CJ, Janssen PA: Cocaine cue in rats as it relates to subjective drug effects: a preliminary report. Eur J Pharmacol 40:195–199, 1976

Comer SD, Haney M, Foltin RW, et al: Amphetamine self-administration by humans: modulation by contingencies associated with task performance. Psychopharmacology (Berl) 127:39–46, 1996

Comer SD, Hart CL, Ward AS, et al: Effects of repeated oral methamphetamine administration in humans. Psychopharmacology (Berl) 155:397–404, 2001

Comer SD, Ashworth JB, Foltin RW, et al: The role of human drug self-administration procedures in the development of medications. Drug Alcohol Depend 96:1–15, 2008

Cook CD, Carroll FI, Beardsley PM: RTI 113, a 3-phenyltropane analog, produces long-lasting cocaine-like discriminative stimulus effects in rats and squirrel monkeys. Eur J Pharmacol 442:93–98, 2002

Cook CE, Jeffcoat AR, Sadler BM, et al: Pharmacokinetics of oral methamphetamine and effects of repeated daily dosing in humans. Drug Metab Dispos 20:856–862, 1992

Cook CE, Jeffcoat AR, Hill JM, et al: Pharmacokinetics of methamphetamine self-administered to human subjects by smoking S-(+)-methamphetamine hydrochloride. Drug Metab Dispos 21:717–723, 1993

Cornish JL, Kalivas PW: Glutamate transmission in the nucleus accumbens mediates relapse in cocaine addiction. J Neurosci 20:RC89, 2000

Craddock D: Anorectic drugs: use in general practice. Drugs 11:378–393, 1976

Crits-Christoph P, Newberg A, Wintering N, et al: Dopamine transporter levels in cocaine dependent subjects. Drug Alcohol Depend 98:70–76, 2008

Cruickshank CC, Montebello ME, Dyer KR, et al: A placebo-controlled trial of mirtazapine for the management of methamphetamine withdrawal. Drug Alcohol Rev 27:326–333, 2008

Cunningham JK, Liu L, Callaghan R: Impact of US and Canadian precursor regulation on methamphetamine purity in the United States. Addiction 104:441–453, 2009

Cunningham KA, Bubar MJ, Anastasio NC: The serotonin 5-HT2C receptor in medial prefrontal cortex exerts rheostatic control over the motivational salience of cocaine-associated cues: new observations from preclinical animal research. Neuropsychopharmacology 35:2319–2321, 2010

Czuchlewski DR, Brackney M, Ewers C, et al: Clinicopathologic features of agranulocytosis in the setting of levamisole-tainted cocaine. Am J Clin Pathol 133:466–472, 2010

Dackis CA, Lynch KG, Yu E, et al: Modafinil and cocaine: a double-blind, placebo-controlled drug interaction study. Drug Alcohol Depend 70:29–37, 2003

Dackis CA, Kampman KM, Lynch KG, et al: A double-blind, placebo-controlled trial of modafinil for cocaine dependence. Neuropsychopharmacology 30:205–211, 2005

Dalley JW, Fryer TD, Brichard L, et al: Nucleus accumbens D2/3 receptors predict trait impulsivity and cocaine reinforcement. Science 315:1267–1270, 2007

Danbolt NC: Glutamate uptake. Prog Neurobiol 65:1–105, 2001

Darracq L, Blanc G, Glowinski J, et al: Importance of the noradrenaline-dopamine coupling in the locomotor activating effects of D-amphetamine. J Neurosci 18:2729–2739, 1998

Degenhardt L, Singleton J, Calabria B, et al: Mortality among cocaine users: a systematic review of cohort studies. Drug Alcohol Depend 113:88–95, 2011

De La Garza R [2nd], Johanson CE: The discriminative stimulus properties of cocaine and d-amphetamine: the effects of three routes of administration. Pharmacol Biochem Behav 24:765–768, 1986

De La Garza R 2nd, Mahoney JJ 3rd, Culbertson C, et al: The acetylcholinesterase inhibitor rivastigmine does not alter total choices for methamphetamine, but may reduce positive subjective effects, in a laboratory model of intravenous self-administration in human volunteers. Pharmacol Biochem Behav 89:200–208, 2008a

De La Garza R [2nd], Shoptaw S, Newton TF: Evaluation of the cardiovascular and subjective effects of rivastigmine in combination with methamphetamine in methamphetamine-dependent human volunteers. Int J Neuropsychopharmacol 11:729–741, 2008b

De La Garza R 2nd, Zorick T, London ED, et al: Evaluation of modafinil effects on cardiovascular, subjective, and reinforcing effects of methamphetamine in methamphetamine-dependent volunteers. Drug Alcohol Depend 106:173–180, 2010

Deminiere JM, Piazza PV, Le Moal M, et al: Experimental approach to individual vulnerability to psychostimulant addiction. Neurosci Biobehav Rev 13:141–147, 1989

Deroche-Gamonet V, Belin D, Piazza PV: Evidence for addiction-like behavior in the rat. Science 305:1014–1017, 2004

Devoto P, Flore G, Pani L, et al: Evidence for co-release of noradrenaline and dopamine from noradrenergic neurons in the cerebral cortex. Mol Psychiatry 6:657–664, 2001

Devoto P, Flore G, Saba P, et al: Co-release of noradrenaline and dopamine in the cerebral cortex elicited by single train and repeated train stimulation of the locus coeruleus. BMC Neurosci 6:31, 2005

de Wit H, Stewart J: Reinstatement of cocaine-reinforced responding in the rat. Psychopharmacology (Berl) 75:134–143, 1981

Di Chiara G, Imperato A: Drugs abused by humans preferentially increase synaptic dopamine concentrations in the mesolimbic system of freely moving rats. Proc Natl Acad Sci U S A 85:5274–5278, 1988

Diercks DB, Fonarow GC, Kirk J, et al: Illicit stimulant use in a United States heart failure population presenting to the emergency department (from the Acute Decompensated Heart Failure National Registry Emergency Module). Am J Cardiol 102:1216–1219, 2008

Ding Y, Singhal T, Planeta-Wilson B, et al: PET imaging of the effects of age and cocaine on the norepinephrine transporter in the human brain using (S,S)-[(11)C]O-methylreboxetine and HRRT. Synapse 64:30–38, 2010

Dinieri JA, Nemeth CL, Parsegian A, et al: Altered sensitivity to rewarding and aversive drugs in mice with inducible disruption of cAMP response element-binding protein function within the nucleus accumbens. J Neurosci 29:1855–1859, 2009

Dobkin C, Nicosia N: The war on drugs: methamphetamine, public health, and crime. Am Econ Rev 99:324–349, 2009

Driscoll RC, Barr FS, Gragg BJ, et al: Determination of therapeutic blood levels of methamphetamine and pentobarbital by GC. J Pharm Sci 60:1492–1495, 1971

Drouin C, Darracq L, Trovero F, et al: Alpha1b-adrenergic receptors control locomotor and rewarding effects of psychostimulants and opiates. J Neurosci 22:2873–2884, 2002

Drug Enforcement Administration (DEA), Department of Justice: Elimination of exemptions for chemical mixtures containing the list I chemicals ephedrine and/or pseudoephedrine. Final rule. Fed Regist 73:39611–39614, 2008

Elkashef AM, Rawson RA, Anderson AL, et al: Bupropion for the treatment of methamphetamine dependence. Neuropsychopharmacology 33:1162–1170, 2008

Ellinwood EH, Balster RL: Rating the behavioral effects of amphetamine. Eur J Pharmacol 28:35–41, 1974

El-Seedi HR, De Smet PA, Beck O, et al: Prehistoric peyote use: alkaloid analysis and radiocarbon dating of archaeological specimens of *Lophophora* from Texas. J Ethnopharmacol 101:238–242, 2005

Erb S, Shaham Y, Stewart J: Stress reinstates cocaine-seeking behavior after prolonged extinction and a drug-free period. Psychopharmacology 128:408–412, 1996

Ernst T, Chang L: Adaptation of brain glutamate plus glutamine during abstinence from chronic methamphetamine use. J Neuroimmune Pharmacol 3:165–172, 2008

Evans SM, Cone EJ, Henningfield JE: Arterial and venous cocaine plasma concentrations in humans: relationship to route of administration, cardiovascular effects and subjective effects. J Psychopharmacol Exp Ther 279:1345–1356, 1996

Everitt BJ, Robbins TW: Neural systems of reinforcement for drug addiction: from actions to habits to compulsion. Nat Neurosci 8:1481–1489, 2005

Evrard I, Legleye S, Cadet-Taïrou A: Composition, purity and perceived quality of street cocaine in France. Int J Drug Policy 21:399–406, 2010

Eyerman DJ, Yamamoto BK: A rapid oxidation and persistent decrease in the vesicular monoamine transporter 2 after methamphetamine. J Neurochem 103:1219–1227, 2007

Ferraro L, Antonelli T, O'Connor WT, et al: The antinarcoleptic drug modafinil increases glutamate release in thalamic areas and hippocampus. Neuroreport 8:2883–2887, 1997

Ferris MJ, Mateo Y, Roberts DC, et al: Cocaine-insensitive dopamine transporters with intact substrate transport produced by self-administration. Biol Psychiatry 69:201–207, 2011

Filip M, Alenina N, Bader M, et al: Behavioral evidence for the significance of serotoninergic (5-HT) receptors in cocaine addiction. Addict Biol 15:227–249, 2010

Fischer J, Cho A: Chemical release of dopamine from striatal homogenates: evidence for an exchange diffusion model. J Pharmacol Exp Ther 208:203–209, 1979

Fischman MW, Schuster CR: Tolerance development to chronic methamphetamine intoxication in the rhesus monkey. Pharmacol Biochem Behav 2:503–508, 1974

Fischman MW, Schuster CR: Cocaine self-administration in humans. Fed Proc 41:241–246, 1982

Fischman MW, Schuster CR, Resnekov L, et al: Cardiovascular and subjective effects of intravenous cocaine administration in humans. Arch Gen Psychiatry 33:983–989, 1976

Fitzgerald LW, Ortiz J, Hamedani AG, et al: Drugs of abuse and stress increase the expression of GluR1 and NMDAR1 glutamate receptor subunits in the rat ventral tegmental area: common adaptations among cross-sensitizing agents. J Neurosci 16:274–282, 1996

Fleckenstein AE, Metzger RR, Beyeler ML, et al: Oxygen radicals diminish dopamine transporter function in rat striatum. Eur J Pharmacol 334:111–114, 1997

Fleckenstein AE, Volz TJ, Riddle EL, et al: New insights into the mechanism of action of amphetamines. Annu Rev Pharmacol Toxicol 47:681–698, 2007

Flores G, Wood GK, Barbeau D, et al: Lewis and Fischer rats: a comparison of dopamine transporter and receptor levels. Brain Res 814:34–40, 1998

Foltin RW, Fischman MW: Smoked and intravenous cocaine in humans: acute tolerance, cardiovascular and subjective effects. J Pharmacol Exp Ther 257:247–261, 1991

Foltin RW, Fischman MW: Self-administration of cocaine by humans: choice between smoked and intravenous cocaine. J Pharmacol Exp Ther 261:841–849, 1992

Foltin RW, Haney M: Intranasal cocaine in humans: acute tolerance, cardiovascular and subjective effects. Pharmacol Biochem Behav 78:93–101, 2004

Foltin RW, Ward AS, Haney M, et al: The effects of escalating doses of smoked cocaine in humans. Drug Alcohol Depend 70:149–157, 2003

Fornai F, Alessandri MG, Torracca MT, et al: Noradrenergic modulation of methamphetamine-induced striatal dopamine depletion. Ann N Y Acad Sci 844:166–177, 1998

Fowler JS, Volkow ND, Wang GJ, et al: [(11)]Cocaine: PET studies of cocaine pharmacokinetics, dopamine transporter availability and dopamine transporter occupancy. Nucl Med Biol 28:561–572, 2001

Fowler JS, Volkow ND, Logan J, et al: Fast uptake and long-lasting binding of methamphetamine in the human brain: comparison with cocaine. Neuroimage 43:756–763, 2008

Freud S, Byck R: The Cocaine Papers. New York, Plume, 1975

Frohmader KS, Pitchers KK, Balfour ME, et al: Mixing pleasures: review of the effects of drugs on sex behavior in humans and animal models. Horm Behav 58:149–162, 2010

Fucci N, De Giovanni N: Adulterants encountered in the illicit cocaine market. Forensic Sci Int 95:247–252, 1998

Fukami G, Hashimoto K, Koike K, et al: Effect of antioxidant N-acetyl-L-cysteine on behavioral changes and neurotoxicity in rats after administration of methamphetamine. Brain Res 1016:90–95, 2004

Gaedcke F: Ueber das Erythroxylin, dargestellt aus den Blättern des in Südamerika cultivirten Strauches Erythroxylon Coca Lam. Arch der Pharm (Weinheim) 132:141–150, 1855

Galanter M, Kleber HD (eds): The American Psychiatric Publishing Textbook of Substance Abuse Treatment, 4th Edition. Washington, DC, American Psychiatric Publishing, 2008

Galea E, Heneka MT, Dello Russo C, et al: Intrinsic regulation of brain inflammatory responses. Cell Mol Neurobiol 23:625–635, 2003

Gass JT, Osborne MP, Watson NL, et al: mGluR5 antagonism attenuates methamphetamine reinforcement and prevents reinstatement of methamphetamine-seeking behavior in rats. Neuropsychopharmacology 34:820–833, 2009

Gawin FH, Kleber HD: Abstinence symptomatology and psychiatric diagnosis in cocaine abusers. Clinical observations. Arch Gen Psychiatry 43:107–113, 1986

Glowinski J, Iversen LL: Regional studies of catecholamines in the rat brain, I: the disposition of [3H]norepinephrine, [3H]dopamine and [3H]dopa in various regions of the brain. J Neurochem 13:655–669, 1966

Gold LH, Balster RL: Evaluation of the cocaine-like discriminative stimulus effects and reinforcing effects of modafinil. Psychopharmacology (Berl) 126:286–292, 1996

Goldberg MF: Cocaine: the first local anesthetic and the "third scourge of humanity": a centennial melodrama. Arch Ophthalmol 102:1443–1447, 1984

Gorelova N, Yang CR: The course of neural projection from the prefrontal cortex to the nucleus accumbens in the rat. Neuroscience 76:689–706, 1997

Grabowski J, Rhoades H, Schmitz J, et al: Dextroamphetamine for cocaine-dependence treatment: a double-blind randomized clinical trial. J Clin Psychopharmacol 21:522–526, 2001

Grabowski J, Rhoades H, Stotts A, et al: Agonist-like or antagonist-like treatment for cocaine dependence with methadone for heroin dependence: two double-blind randomized clinical trials. Neuropsychopharmacology 29:969–981, 2004

Graves SM, Napier TC: Mirtazapine alters cue-associated methamphetamine seeking in rats. Biol Psychiatry 69:275–281, 2011

Greenwald G: Drug decriminalization in Portugal: lessons for creating fair and successful drug policies. Cato Institute White Paper, April 2, 2009. Available at: http://www.cato.org/pub_display.php?pub_id=10080. Accessed March 16, 2011.

Haile CN: Neurochemical and neurobehavioral consequences of methamphetamine abuse, in Drug Abuse Handbook, 2nd Edition. Edited by Karch SB. Boca Raton, FL, CRC Press, 2007, pp 478–503

Haile CN, Kosten TA: Differential effects of D1- and D2-like compounds on cocaine self-administration in Lewis and Fischer 344 inbred rats. J Psychopharmacol Exp Ther 299:509–518, 2001

Haile CN, During MJ, Jatlow PI, et al: Disulfiram facilitates the development and expression of locomotor sensitization to cocaine in rats. Biol Psychiatry 54:915–921, 2003

Haile CN, Kosten TR, Kosten TA: Genetics of dopamine and its contribution to cocaine addiction. Behav Genet 37:119–145, 2007

Haile CN, Kosten TR, Kosten TA: Pharmacogenetic treatments for drug addiction: cocaine, amphetamine and methamphetamine. Am J Drug Alcohol Abuse 35:161–177, 2009

Haile CN, De La Garza R 2nd, Newton T: Methamphetamine cured my cocaine addiction. J Addict Res Ther 1:103, 2010

Hameedi FA, Rosen MI, McCance-Katz EF, et al: Behavioral, physiological, and pharmacological interaction of cocaine and disulfiram in humans. Biol Psychiatry 37:560–563, 1995

Harris DS, Boxenbaum H, Everhart ET, et al: The bioavailability of intranasal and smoked methamphetamine. Clin Pharmacol Ther 74:475–486, 2003. doi:10.1016/j.clpt.2003.08.002

Harris JE, Baldessarini RJ: Uptake of (3H)-catecholamines by homogenates of rat corpus striatum and cerebral cortex: effects of amphetamine analogues. Neuropharmacology 12:669–679, 1973

Hart CL, Ward AS, Haney M, et al: Methamphetamine self-administration by humans. Psychopharmacology (Berl) 157:75–81, 2001

Hart CL, Gunderson EW, Perez K, et al: Acute physiological and behavioral effects of intranasal methamphetamine in humans. Neuropsychopharmacology 33:1847–1855, 2008a

Hart CL, Haney M, Vosburg SK, et al: Smoked cocaine self-administration is decreased by modafinil. Neuropsychopharmacology 33:761–768, 2008b

Hashimoto K, Tsukada H, Nishiyama S, et al: Protective effects of N-acetyl-L-cysteine
on the reduction of dopamine transporters in the striatum of monkeys treated
with methamphetamine. Neuropsychopharmacology 29:2018–2023, 2004

Hashimoto K, Tsukada H, Nishiyama S, et al: Protective effects of minocycline on the
reduction of dopamine transporters in the striatum after administration of methamphetamine: a positron emission tomography study in conscious monkeys.
Biol Psychiatry 61:577–581, 2007

Hassel B, Boldingh KA, Narvensen C, et al: Glutamate transport, glutamine syn-
thetase and phosphate-activated glutaminase in rat CNS white matter. A quantitative study. J Neurochem 87:230–237, 2003

Hawks RL, Kopin IJ, Colburn RW, et al: Norcocaine: a pharmacologically active metabolite of cocaine found in brain. Life Sci 15:2189–2195, 1974

Heinzerling KG, Swanson AN, Kim S, et al: Randomized, double-blind, placebo-
controlled trial of modafinil for the treatment of methamphetamine dependence.
Drug Alcohol Depend 109:20–29, 2010

Herin DV, Rush CR, Grabowski J: Agonist-like pharmacotherapy for stimulant dependence: preclinical, human laboratory, and clinical studies. Ann N Y Acad Sci
1187:76–100, 2010

Higashi H, Inanaga K, Nishi S, et al: Enhancement of dopamine actions on rat nucleus
accumbens neurones in vitro after methamphetamine pre-treatment. J Physiol
408:587–603, 1989

Holtmaat AJ, Trachtenberg JT, Wilbrecht L, et al: Transient and persistent dendritic
spines in the neocortex in vivo. Neuron 45:279–291, 2005

Imam SZ, Ali SF: Selenium, an antioxidant, attenuates methamphetamine-induced
dopaminergic toxicity and peroxynitrite generation. Brain Res 855:186–191,
2000

Imam SZ, Newport GD, Islam F, et al: Selenium, an antioxidant, protects against
methamphetamine-induced dopaminergic neurotoxicity. Brain Res 18:575–578,
1999

Imbesi M, Uz T, Manev R, et al: Minocycline increases phosphorylation and membrane insertion of neuronal GluR1 receptors. Neurosci Lett 447:134–137, 2008

Indriati E, Buikstra JE: Coca chewing in prehistoric coastal Peru: dental evidence. Am
J Phys Anthropol 114:242–257, 2001

Iso Y, Grajkowska E, Wroblewski JT, et al: Synthesis and structure-activity relationships of 3-[(2-methyl-1,3-thiazol-4-yl)ethynyl]pyridine analogues as potent,
noncompetitive metabotropic glutamate receptor subtype 5 antagonists: search
for cocaine medications. J Med Chem 49:1080–1100, 2006

Iyo M, Sekine Y, Mori N: Neuromechanism of developing methamphetamine psychosis: a neuroimaging study. Ann N Y Acad Sci 1025:288–295, 2004

Jasinski DR, Kovacevi-Ristanovi R: Evaluation of the abuse liability of modafinil and
other drugs for excessive daytime sleepiness associated with narcolepsy. Clin
Neuropharmacol 23:149–156, 2000

Jasinski DR, Krishnan S: Abuse liability and safety of oral lisdexamfetamine dimesyl-
ate in individuals with a history of stimulant abuse. J Psychopharmacol 23:419–
427, 2009

Jatlow P: Cocaine: analysis, pharmacokinetics, and metabolic disposition. Yale J Biol
Med 61:105–113, 1988

Javaid JI, Fischman MW, Schuster CR, et al: Cocaine plasma concentration: relation to physiological and subjective effects in humans. Science 202:227–228, 1978

Johanson CE, Balster RL, Bonese K: Self-administration of psychomotor stimulant drugs: the effects of unlimited access. Pharmacol Biochem Behav 4:45–51, 1976

Johanson CE, Lundahl LH, Lockhart N, et al: Intravenous cocaine discrimination in humans. Exp Clin Psychopharmacol 14:99–108, 2006

Kalechstein AD, Newton TF, Green M: Methamphetamine dependence is associated with neurocognitive impairment in the initial phases of abstinence. J Neuropsychiatry Clin Neurosci 15:215–220, 2003

Kalechstein AD, De La Garza 2nd, Newton TF, et al: Quantitative EEG abnormalities are associated with memory impairment in recently abstinent methamphetamine-dependent individuals. J Neuropsychiatry Clin Neurosci 21:254–258, 2009

Kalechstein AD, De La Garza R 2nd, Newton TF: Modafinil administration improves working memory in methamphetamine-dependent individuals who demonstrate baseline impairment. Am J Addict 19:340–344, 2010

Kalivas PW: The glutamate homeostasis hypothesis of addiction. Nat Rev Neurosci 10:561–572, 2009

Kalivas PW, McFarland K: Brain circuitry and the reinstatement of cocaine-seeking behavior. Psychopharmacology (Berl) 168:44–56, 2003

Kalivas PW, McFarland K, Bowers S, et al: Glutamate transmission and addiction to cocaine. Ann N Y Acad Sci 1003:169–175, 2003

Kamata K, Rebec GV: Long-term amphetamine treatment attenuates or reverses the depression of neuronal activity produced by dopamine agonists in the ventral tegmental area. Life Sci 34:2419–2427, 1984

Kamien JB, Bickel WK, Hughes JR, et al: Drug discrimination by humans compared to nonhumans: current status and future directions. Psychopharmacology (Berl) 111:259–270, 1993

Káradóttir R, Cavelier P, Bergersen LH, et al: NMDA receptors are expressed in oligo-dendrocytes and activated in ischaemia. Nature 438:1162–1166, 2005

Karila L, Weinstein A, Aubin HJ, et al: Pharmacological approaches to methamphetamine dependence: a focused review. Br J Clin Pharmacol 69:578–592, 2010

Katz JL, Higgins ST: The validity of the reinstatement model of craving and relapse to drug use. Psychopharmacology (Berl) 168:21–30, 2003

Katz JL, Sharpe LG, Jaffe JH, et al: Discriminative stimulus effects of inhaled cocaine in squirrel monkeys. Psychopharmacology (Berl) 105:317–321, 1991

Kau KS, Madayag A, Mantsch JR, et al: Blunted cystine-glutamate antiporter function in the nucleus accumbens promotes cocaine-induced drug seeking. Neuroscience 155:530–537, 2008

Kil HY, Zhang J, Piantadosi CA: Brain temperature alters hydroxyl radical production during cerebral ischemia/reperfusion in rats. J Cereb Blood Flow Metab 16:100–106, 1996

Kim D, Roh S, Kim Y, et al: High concentrations of plasma brain-derived neurotrophic factor in methamphetamine users. Neurosci Lett 388:112–115, 2005

Kiyatkin EA, Sharma HS: Acute methamphetamine intoxication brain hyperthermia, blood-brain barrier, brain edema, and morphological cell abnormalities. Int Rev Neurobiol 88:65–100, 2009a

Kiyatkin EA, Sharma HS: Permeability of the blood-brain barrier depends on brain temperature. Neuroscience 161:926–939, 2009b

Kleven MS, Anthony EW, Woolverton WL: Pharmacological characterization of the discriminative stimulus effects of cocaine in rhesus monkeys. J Psychopharmacol Exp Ther 254:312–317, 1990

Knackstedt LA, Kalivas PW: Glutamate and reinstatement. Curr Opin Pharmacol 9:59–64, 2009

Knackstedt LA, Moussawi K, Lalumiere R, et al: Extinction training after cocaine self-administration induces glutamatergic plasticity to inhibit cocaine seeking. J Neurosci 30:7984–7992, 2010

Kolbrich EA, Barnes AJ, Gorelick DA, et al: Major and minor metabolites of cocaine in human plasma following controlled subcutaneous cocaine administration. J Anal Toxicol 30:501–510, 2006

Kongsakon R, Papadopoulos KI, Saguansiritham R: Mirtazapine in amphetamine detoxification: a placebo-controlled pilot study. Int Clin Psychopharmacol 20:253–256, 2005

Koob GF, Volkow ND: Neurocircuitry of addiction. Neuropsychopharmacology 35:217–238, 2010

Kornetsky C, Esposito RU: Euphorigenic drugs: effects on the reward pathways of the brain. Fed Proc 38:2473–2476, 1979

Krasnova IN, Cadet JL: Methamphetamine toxicity and messengers of death. Brain Res Rev 60:379–407, 2009

lanacion.com. (2010, April 16). Bolivia lanza la Coca Colla. April 16, 2010. Available at: http://www.lanacion.com.ar/1254929. Accessed June 26, 2011.

LaRowe SD, Markidian P, Malcolm R, et al: Safety and tolerability of N-acetylcysteine in cocaine-dependent individuals. Am J Addict 15:105–110, 2006

LaRowe SD, Myrick H, Hedden S, et al: Is cocaine desire reduced by N-acetylcysteine? Am J Psychiatry 164:1115–1117, 2007

Laruelle M, Gelernter J, Innis RB: D2 receptors binding potential is not affected by Taq1 polymorphism at the D2 receptor gene. Mol Psychiatry 3:261–265, 1998

Lategan AJ, Marien MR, Colpaert FC: Effects of locus coeruleus lesions on the release of endogenous dopamine in the rat nucleus accumbens and caudate nucleus as determined by intracerebral microdialysis. Brain Res 523:134–138, 1990

Lathers CM, Charles JB: Orthostatic hypotension in patients, bed rest subjects, and astronauts. J Clin Pharmacol 34:403–417, 1994

LaVoie MJ, Hastings TG: Dopamine quinone formation and protein modification associated with the striatal neurotoxicity of methamphetamine: evidence against a role for extracellular dopamine. J Neurosci 19:1484–1491, 1999

Lee B, Platt DM, Rowlett JK, et al: Attenuation of behavioral effects of cocaine by the metabotropic glutamate receptor 5 antagonist 2-methyl-6-(phenylethynyl)-pyridine in squirrel monkeys: comparison with dizocilpine. J Psychopharmacol Exp Ther 312:1232–1240, 2005

Lee KW, Kim Y, Kim AM, et al: Cocaine-induced dendritic spine formation in D1 and D2 dopamine receptor-containing medium spiny neurons in nucleus accumbens. Proc Natl Acad Sci U S A 103:3399–3404, 2006

Le Foll B, Diaz J, Sokoloff P: A single cocaine exposure increases BDNF and D3 receptor expression: implications for drug-conditioning. Neuroreport 16:175–178, 2005

Lewis DA, Melchitzky DS, Sesack SR, et al: Dopamine transporter immunoreactivity in monkey cerebral cortex: regional, laminar, and ultrastructural localization. J Comp Neurol 432:119–136, 2001

Li S, Campbell BL, Katz JL: Interactions of cocaine with dopamine uptake inhibitors or dopamine releasers in rats discriminating cocaine. J Psychopharmacol Exp Ther 317:1088–1096, 2006

Lile JA, Stoops WW, Glaser PE, et al: Discriminative stimulus, subject-rated and cardiovascular effects of cocaine alone and in combination with aripiprazole in humans. J Psychopharmacol October 15, 2010 [Epub ahead of print]

Liu Y, Edwards RH: The role of vesicular transport proteins in synaptic transmission and neural degeneration. Annu Rev Neurosci 20:125–156, 1997

Mack F, Bönisch H: Dissociation constants and lipophilicity of catecholamines and related compounds. Naunyn Schmiedebergs Arch Pharmacol 310:1–9, 1979

Mack RB: The iceman cometh and killeth: smokable methamphetamine. N C Med J 51:276–278, 1990

Madayag A, Lobner D, Kau KS, et al: Repeated N-acetylcysteine administration alters plasticity-dependent effects of cocaine. J Neurosci 27:13968–13976, 2007

Madras BK, Xie Z, Lin Z, et al: Modafinil occupies dopamine and norepinephrine transporters in vivo and modulates the transporters and trace amine activity in vitro. J Psychopharmacol Exp Ther 319:561–569, 2006

Mahoney JJ 3rd, Hawkins RY, De La Garza 2nd, et al: Relationship between gender and psychotic symptoms in cocaine-dependent and methamphetamine-dependent participants. Gend Med 7:414–421, 2010

Maldonado R, Saiardi A, Valverde O, et al: Absence of opiate rewarding effects in mice lacking dopamine D2 receptors. Nature 388:586–589, 1997

Mancini MA, Linhorst DM: Harm reduction in community mental health settings. J Soc Work Disabil Rehabil 9:130–147, 2010

Mardikian PN, LaRowe SD, Hedden S, et al: An open-label trial of N-acetylcysteine for the treatment of cocaine dependence: a pilot study. Prog Neuropsychopharmacol Biol Psychiatry 31:389–394, 2007

Markou A, Weiss F, Gold LH, et al: Animal models of drug craving. Psychopharmacology (Berl) 112:163–182, 1993

Marshall BD, Werb D: Health outcomes associated with methamphetamine use among young people: a systematic review. Addiction 105:991–1002, 2010

Martin WR, Sloan JW, Sapira JD, et al: Physiologic, subjective, and behavioral effects of amphetamine, methamphetamine, ephedrine, phenmetrazine, and methylphenidate in man. Clin Pharmacol Ther 12:245–258, 1971

Martinez D, Broft A, Foltin RW, et al: Cocaine dependence and d2 receptor availability in the functional subdivisions of the striatum: relationship with cocaine-seeking behavior. Neuropsychopharmacology 29:1190–1202, 2004

Martinez D, Narendran R, Foltin RW, et al: Amphetamine-induced dopamine release: markedly blunted in cocaine dependence and predictive of the choice to self-administer cocaine. Am J Psychiatry 164:622–629, 2007

Martinez D, Greene K, Broft A, et al: Lower level of endogenous dopamine in patients with cocaine dependence: findings from PET imaging of D(2)/D(3) receptors following acute dopamine depletion. Am J Psychiatry 166:1170–1177, 2009

Matsuzaki M, Honkura N, Ellis-Davies GC, et al: Structural basis of long-term potentiation in single dendritic spines. Nature 429:761–766, 2004

McBean GJ: Cerebral cystine uptake: a tale of two transporters. Trends Pharmacol Sci 23:299–302, 2002

McCann UD, Wong DF, Yokoi F, et al: Reduced striatal dopamine transporter density in abstinent methamphetamine and methcathinone users: evidence from positron emission tomography studies with [11C]WIN-35,428. J Neurosci 18:8417–8422, 1998

McElhiney MC, Rabkin JG, Rabkin R, et al: Provigil (modafinil) plus cognitive behavioral therapy for methamphetamine use in HIV+ gay men: a pilot study. Am J Drug Alcohol Abuse 35:34–37, 2009

McFarland K, Lapish CC, Kalivas PW: Prefrontal glutamate release into the core of the nucleus accumbens mediates cocaine-induced reinstatement of drug-seeking behavior. J Neurosci 23:3531–3537, 2003

McGaugh J, Mancino MJ, Feldman Z, et al: Open-label pilot study of modafinil for methamphetamine dependence. J Clin Psychopharmacol 29:488–491, 2009

McGregor C, Srisurapanont M, Mitchell A, et al: Symptoms and sleep patterns during inpatient treatment of methamphetamine withdrawal: a comparison of mirtazapine and modafinil with treatment as usual. J Subst Abuse Treat 35:334–342, 2008

McKenna ML, Ho BT: The role of dopamine in the discriminative stimulus properties of cocaine. Neuropharmacology 19:297–303, 1980

McKinney CD, Postiglione KF, Herold DA: Benzocaine-adultered street cocaine in association with methemoglobinemia. Clin Chem 38:596–597, 1992

Melega WP, Laan G, Harvey DC, et al: Methamphetamine increases basal ganglia iron to levels observed in aging. Neuroreport 18:1741–1745, 2007

Metzger RR, Haughey HM, Wilkins DG, et al: Methamphetamine-induced rapid decrease in dopamine transporter function: role of dopamine and hyperthermia. J Pharmacol Exp Ther 295:1077–1085, 2000

Miller DB, O'Callaghan JP: Environment-, drug- and stress-induced alterations in body temperature affect the neurotoxicity of substituted amphetamines in the C57BL/6J mouse. J Psychopharmacol Exp Ther 270:752–760, 1994

Miner LH, Schroeter S, Blakely RD, et al: Ultrastructural localization of the norepinephrine transporter in superficial and deep layers of the rat prelimbic prefrontal cortex and its spatial relationship to probable dopamine terminals. J Comp Neurol 466:478–494, 2003

Mitchell HA, Weinshenker D: Good night and good luck: norepinephrine in sleep pharmacology. Biochem Pharmacol 79:801–809, 2010

Mooney ME, Schmitz JM, Moeller FG, et al: Safety, tolerability and efficacy of levodopa-carbidopa treatment for cocaine dependence: two double-blind, randomized, clinical trials. Drug Alcohol Depend 88:214–223, 2007

Mooney ME, Herin DV, Schmitz JM, et al: Effects of oral methamphetamine on cocaine use: a randomized, double-blind, placebo-controlled trial. Drug Alcohol Depend 101:34–41, 2009

Moran MM, McFarland K, Melendez RI, et al: Cystine/glutamate exchange regulates metabotropic glutamate receptor presynaptic inhibition of excitatory transmission and vulnerability to cocaine seeking. J Neurosci 25:6389–6393, 2005

Morón JA, Brockington A, Wise A, et al: Dopamine uptake through the norepinephrine transporter in brain regions with low levels of the dopamine transporter: evidence from knock-out mouse lines. J Neurosci 22:389–395, 2002

Morrison JH, Molliver ME, Grzanna R, et al: The intra-cortical trajectory of the coeruleo-cortical projection in the rat: a tangentially organized cortical afferent. Neuroscience 6:139–158, 1981

Moussawi K, Pacchioni A, Moran M, et al: N-Acetylcysteine reverses cocaine-induced metaplasticity. Nat Neurosci 12:182–189, 2009

Moussawi K, Zhou W, Shen H, et al: Reversing cocaine-induced synaptic potentiation provides enduring protection from relapse. Proc Natl Acad Sci U S A 108:385–390, 2011

Muntaner C, Kumor KM, Magoshi C, et al: Intravenous cocaine infusions in humans: dose responsivity and correlations of cardiovascular vs. subjective effects. Pharmacol Biochem Behav 34:697–703, 1989

Nägerl UV, Eberhorn N, Cambridge SB, et al: Bidirectional activity-dependent morphological plasticity in hippocampal neurons. Neuron 44:759–767, 2004

Narendran R, Frankle WG, Mason NS, et al: Positron emission tomography imaging of amphetamine-induced dopamine release in the human cortex: a comparative evaluation of the high affinity dopamine D2/3 radiotracers [11C]FLB 457 and [11C]fallypride. Synapse 63:447–461, 2009

Narita M, Aoki K, Tagaki M, et al: Implication of brain-derived neurotrophic factor in the release of dopamine and dopamine-related behaviors induced by methamphetamine. Neuroscience 119:767–775, 2003

National Drug Intelligence Center: National methamphetamine threat assessment. 2009. Available at: http://www.justice.gov/ndic/pubs32/32166/32166p.pdf. Accessed March 17, 2011.

Negus SS, Mello NK: Effects of chronic d-amphetamine treatment on cocaine- and food-maintained responding under a second-order schedule in rhesus monkeys. Drug Alcohol Depend 70:39–52, 2003

Negus SS, Mello NK, Blough BE, et al: Monoamine releasers with varying selectivity for dopamine/norepinephrine versus serotonin release as candidate "agonist" medications for cocaine dependence: studies in assays of cocaine discrimination and cocaine self-administration in rhesus monkeys. J Psychopharmacol Exp Ther 320:627–636, 2007

Nestler EJ: Common molecular and cellular substrates of addiction and memory. Neurobiol Learn Mem 78:637–647, 2002

Nestler EJ: Is there a common molecular pathway for addiction? Nat Neurosci 8:1445–1449, 2005

Newman JL, Carroll ME: Reinforcing effects of smoked methamphetamine in rhesus monkeys. Psychopharmacology (Berl) 188:193–200, 2006

Newton TF, Ling W, Kalechstein AD, et al: Risperidone pre-treatment reduces the euphoric effects of experimentally administered cocaine. Psychiatry Res 102:227–233, 2001

Newton TF, Cook IA, Kalechstein AD, et al: Quantitative EEG abnormalities in recently abstinent methamphetamine dependent individuals. Clin Neurophysiol 114:410–415, 2003

Newton TF, Kalechstein AD, Duran S, et al: Methamphetamine abstinence syndrome: preliminary findings. Am J Addict 13:248–255, 2004

Newton TF, De La Garza 2nd, Kalechstein AD, et al: Cocaine and methamphetamine produce different patterns of subjective and cardiovascular effects. Pharmacol Biochem Behav 82:90–97, 2005a

Newton TF, Roache JD, De La Garza 2nd, et al: Safety of intravenous methamphetamine administration during treatment with bupropion. Psychopharmacology (Berl) 182:426–435, 2005b

Newton TF, Roache JD, De La Garza 2nd, et al: Bupropion reduces methamphet-amine-induced subjective effects and cue-induced craving. Neuropsychophar-macology 31:1537–1544, 2006

The New York Times: How Coca-Cola obtains its coca. July 1, 1988. Available at: http://www.nytimes.com/1988/07/01/business/how-coca-cola-obtains-its-coca.html. Accessed June 26, 2011.

Niemann A: Ueber eine neue organische Base in den Cocablättern. Arch der Pharm (Weinheim) 153:129–155, 1860

Novak M, Halbout B, O'Connor EC, et al: Incentive learning underlying cocaine-seeking requires mGluR5 receptors located on dopamine D1 receptor-express-ing neurons. J Neurosci 30:11973–11982, 2010

Numachi Y, Ohara A, Yamashita M, et al: Methamphetamine-induced hyperthermia and lethal toxicity: role of the dopamine and serotonin transporters. Eur J Phar-macol 572:120–128, 2007

Nutt D, King LA, Saulsbury W, et al: Development of a rational scale to assess the harm of drugs of potential misuse. Lancet 369:1047–1053, 2007

O'Dell SJ, Weihmuller FB, Marshall JF: Methamphetamine-induced dopamine over-flow and injury to striatal dopamine terminals: attenuation by dopamine D1 or D2 antagonists. J Neurochem 60:1792–1799, 1993

Okamoto K, Nagai T, Miyawaki A, et al: Rapid and persistent modulation of actin dy-namics regulates postsynaptic reorganization underlying bidirectional plasticity. Nat Neurosci 7:1104–1112, 2004

Olds J, Milner P: Positive reinforcement produced by electrical stimulation of septal area and other regions of rat brain. J Comp Physiol Psychol 47:419–427, 1954

Oliveto A, Poling J, Mancino MJ, et al: Randomized, double blind, placebo-controlled trial of disulfiram for the treatment of cocaine dependence in methadone-stabi-lized patients. Drug Alcohol Depend 113:184–191, 2011

Olson VG, Zabetian CP, Bolanos CA, et al: Regulation of drug reward by cAMP re-sponse element-binding protein: evidence for two functionally distinct subre-gions of the ventral tegmental area. J Neurosci 25:5553–5562, 2005

O'Neil ML, Kuczenski R, Segal DS, et al: Escalating dose pretreatment induces phar-macodynamic and not pharmacokinetic tolerance to a subsequent high-dose methamphetamine binge. Synapse 60:465–473, 2006

Pacchioni AM, Vallone J, Worley PF, et al: Neuronal pentraxins modulate cocaine-induced neuroadaptations. J Psychopharmacol Exp Ther 328:183–192, 2009

Pacher P, Beckman JS, Liaudet L: Nitric oxide and peroxynitrite in health and disease. Physiol Rev 87:315–424, 2007

Paladini CA, Fiorillo CD, Morikawa H, et al: Amphetamine selectively blocks inhib-itory glutamate transmission in dopamine neurons. Nat Neurosci 4:275–281, 2001

Panlilio LV, Weiss SJ, Schindler CW: Cocaine self-administration increased by com-pounding discriminative stimuli. Psychopharmacology (Berl) 125:202–208, 1996

Parry HJ, Balter MB, Mellinger GD, et al: National patterns of psychotherapeutic drug use. Arch Gen Psychiatry 28:18–74, 1973

Peltier RL, Li DH, Lytle D, et al: Chronic d-amphetamine or methamphetamine pro-duces cross-tolerance to the discriminative and reinforcing stimulus effects of cocaine. J Psychopharmacol Exp Ther 277:212–218, 1996

Pérez-Mañá C, Castells X, Vidal X, et al: Efficacy of indirect dopamine agonists for psychostimulant dependence: a systematic review and meta-analysis of randomized controlled trials. J Subst Abuse Treat 40:109–122, 2011

Perez-Reyes M, White WR, McDonald SA, et al: Clinical effects of daily methamphetamine administration. Clin Neuropharmacol 14:352–358, 1991

Petrakis IL, Carroll KM, Nich C, et al: Disulfiram treatment for cocaine dependence in methadone-maintained opioid addicts. Addiction 95:219–228, 2000

Pettit HO, Justice JB: Dopamine in the nucleus accumbens during cocaine self-administration as studied by in vivo microdialysis. Pharmacol Biochem Behav 34:899–904, 1989

Pettit HO, Ettenberg A, Bloom FE, et al: Destruction of dopamine in the nucleus accumbens selectively attenuates cocaine but not heroin self-administration in rats. Psychopharmacology (Berl) 84:167–173, 1984

Piazza PV, Le Moal M: The role of stress in drug self-administration. Trends Pharmacol Sci 19:67–74, 1998

Pickens R, Meisch RA, Dougherty JA: Chemical interactions in methamphetamine reinforcement. Psychol Rep 23:1267–1270, 1968

Piness G, Miller H, Alles G: Clinical observations on phenylaminoethanol sulphate. JAMA 94:790–791, 1930

Ping A, Xi J, Prasad JM, et al: Contributions of nucleus accumbens core and shell GluR1 containing AMPA receptors in AMPA- and cocaine-primed reinstatement of cocaine-seeking behavior. Brain Res 1215:173–182, 2008

Preseton KL, Wagner GC, Schuster CR, et al: Long-term effects of repeated methylamphetamine administration on monoamine neurons in the rhesus monkey brain. Brain Res 338:243–248, 1985

Ramirez SH, Potula R, Fan S, et al: Methamphetamine disrupts blood-brain barrier function by induction of oxidative stress in brain endothelial cells. J Cereb Blood Flow Metab 29:1933–1945, 2009

Rasmussen N: America's first amphetamine epidemic 1929–1971: a quantitative and qualitative retrospective with implications for the present. Am J Public Health 98:974–985, 2008

Rasmussen N: On Speed: The Many Lives of Amphetamine. New York, New York University Press, 2009

Rau KS, Birdsall E, Hanson JE, et al: Bupropion increases striatal vesicular monoamine transport. Neuropharmacology 49:820–830, 2005

Rawson RA, Marinelli-Casey P, Anglin MD, et al: A multi-site comparison of psychosocial approaches for the treatment of methamphetamine dependence. Addiction 99:708–717, 2004

Reed SC, Haney M, Evans SM, et al: Cardiovascular and subjective effects of repeated smoked cocaine administration in experienced cocaine users. Drug Alcohol Depend 102:102–107, 2009

Reichel CM, See RE: Modafinil effects on reinstatement of methamphetamine seeking in a rat model of relapse. Psychopharmacology (Berl) 210:337–346, 2010

Reiner BC, Keblesh JP, Xiong H: Methamphetamine abuse, HIV infection, and neurotoxicity. Int J Physiol Pathophysiol Pharmacol 1:162–179, 2009

Rescorla RA, Solomon RL: Two-process learning theory: relationships between Pavlovian conditioning and instrumental learning. Psychol Rev 74:151–182, 1967

Riddle EL, Topham MK, Haycock JW, et al: Differential trafficking of the vesicular monoamine transporter-2 by methamphetamine and cocaine. Eur J Pharmacol 449:71–74, 2002

Ritz MC, Lamb RJ, Goldberg SR, et al: Cocaine receptors on dopamine transporters are related to self-administration of cocaine. Science 237:1219–1223, 1987

Rivera MA, Aufderheide AC, Cartmell LW, et al: Antiquity of coca-leaf chewing in the south central Andes: a 3,000 year archaeological record of coca-leaf chewing from northern Chile. J Psychoactive Drugs 37:455–458, 2005

Roberts DC, Koob GF: Disruption of cocaine self-administration following 6-hydroxydopamine lesions of the ventral tegmental area in rats. Pharmacol Biochem Behav 17:901–904, 1982

Robinson TE, Berridge KC: The neural basis of drug craving: an incentive-sensitization theory of addiction. Brain Res Brain Res Rev 18:247–291, 1993

Robinson TE, Kolb B: Persistent structural modifications in nucleus accumbens and prefrontal cortex neurons produced by previous experience with amphetamine. J Neurosci 17:8491–8497, 1997

Robinson TE, Kolb B: Structural plasticity associated with exposure to drugs of abuse. Neuropharmacology 47 (suppl 1):33–46, 2004

Rocha A, Kalivas PW: Role of the prefrontal cortex and nucleus accumbens in reinstating methamphetamine seeking. Eur J Neurosci 31:903–909, 2010

Rocha BA, Fumagalli F, Gainetdinov RR, et al: Cocaine self-administration in dopamine-transporter knockout mice. Nat Neurosci 1:132–137, 1998

Rothman RB, Baumann MH, Dersch CM, et al: Amphetamine-type central nervous system stimulants release norepinephrine more potently than they release dopamine and serotonin. Synapse 39:32–41, 2001

Rothman RB, Blough BE, Baumann MH: Dopamine/serotonin releasers as medications for stimulant addictions. Prog Brain Res 172:385–406, 2008

Rush CR, Kelly TH, Hays LR, et al: Discriminative-stimulus effects of modafinil in cocaine-trained humans. Drug Alcohol Depend 67:311–322, 2002

Rush CR, Stoops WW, Hays LR: Cocaine effects during D-amphetamine maintenance: a human laboratory analysis of safety, tolerability and efficacy. Drug Alcohol Depend 99:261–271, 2009

Rush CR, Stoops WW, Sevak RJ, et al: Cocaine choice in humans during D-amphetamine maintenance. J Clin Psychopharmacol 30:152–159, 2010

Russo SJ, Dietz DM, Dumitriu D, et al: The addicted synapse: mechanisms of synaptic and structural plasticity in nucleus accumbens. Trends Neurosci 33:267–276, 2010

Sailasuta N, Abulseoud O, Harris KC, et al: Glial dysfunction in abstinent methamphetamine abusers. J Cereb Blood Flow Metab 30:950–960, 2010a

Sailasuta N, Abulseoud O, Hernandez M, et al: Metabolic abnormalities in abstinent methamphetamine dependent subjects. Subst Abuse 2010:9–20, 2010b

Salo R, Flower K, Kielstein A, et al: Psychiatric comorbidity in methamphetamine dependence. Psychiatry Res 186:356–361, 2011

Sarti F, Borgland SL, Kharazia VN, et al: Acute cocaine exposure alters spine density and long-term potentiation in the ventral tegmental area. Eur J Neurosci 26:749–756, 2007

Schepers RJF, Oyler JM, Joseph RE Jr, et al: Methamphetamine and amphetamine pharmacokinetics in oral fluid and plasma after controlled oral methamphetamine administration to human volunteers. Clin Chem 49:121–132, 2003

Schmidt HD, Pierce RC: Cocaine-induced neuroadaptations in glutamate transmission: potential therapeutic targets for craving and addiction. Ann N Y Acad Sci 1187:35–75, 2010

Schmitz JM, Mooney ME, Moeller FG, et al: Levodopa pharmacotherapy for cocaine dependence: choosing the optimal behavioral therapy platform. Drug Alcohol Depend 94:142–150, 2008

Schroeder JP, Cooper DA, Schank JR, et al: Disulfiram attenuates drug-primed reinstatement of cocaine seeking via inhibition of dopamine beta-hydroxylase. Neuropsychopharmacology 35:2440–2449, 2010

Schuster CR, Thompson T: Self-administration of and behavioral dependence on drugs. Annu Rev Pharmacol 9:483–502,1969. doi:10.1146/annurev.pa.09.040169 .002411

Schwendt M, Rocha A, See RE, et al: Extended methamphetamine self-administration in rats results in a selective reduction of dopamine transporter levels in the prefrontal cortex and dorsal striatum not accompanied by marked monoaminergic depletion. J Psychopharmacol Exp Ther 331:555–562, 2009

Scott JC, Woods SP, Matt GE, et al: Neurocognitive effects of methamphetamine: a critical review and meta-analysis. Neuropsychol Rev 17:275–297, 2007

Seevers MH, Schuster CR: Self-administration of psychoactive drugs by the monkey: a measure of psychological dependence. Science 158:535, 1967

Sekine Y, Iyo M, Ouchi Y, et al: Methamphetamine-related psychiatric symptoms and reduced brain dopamine transporters studied with PET. Am J Psychiatry 58:1206–1214, 2001

Sesack SR, Carr DB, Omelchenko N, et al: Anatomical substrates for glutamate-dopamine interactions: evidence for specificity of connections and extrasynaptic actions. Ann N Y Acad Sci 1003:36–52, 2003

Sevak RJ, Stoops WW, Hays LR, et al: Discriminative stimulus and subject-rated effects of methamphetamine, d-amphetamine, methylphenidate, and triazolam in methamphetamine-trained humans. J Psychopharmacol Exp Ther 328:1007–1018, 2009

Shaffer H: Classics revisited. Uber Coca. By Sigmund Freud. J Subst Abuse Treat 1:206–217, 1984

Shearer J, Wodak A, van Beek I, et al: Pilot randomized double blind placebo-controlled study of dexamphetamine for cocaine dependence. Addiction 98:1137–1141, 2003

Shearer J, Darke S, Rodgers C, et al: A double-blind, placebo-controlled trial of modafinil (200 mg/day) for methamphetamine dependence. Addiction 104:224–233, 2009

Shen H, Toda S, Moussawi K, et al: Altered dendritic spine plasticity in cocaine-withdrawn rats. J Neurosci 29:2876–2884, 2009

Sheng P, Cerruti C, Ali S, et al: Nitric oxide is a mediator of methamphetamine (METH)-induced neurotoxicity. In vitro evidence from primary cultures of mesencephalic cells. Ann N Y Acad Sci 801:174–186, 1996

Sherer MA, Kumor KM, Jaffe JH: Effects of intravenous cocaine are partially attenuated by haloperidol. Psychiatry Res 27:117–125, 1989

Shi WX, Pun CL, Zhang XX, et al: Dual effects of D-amphetamine on dopamine neurons mediated by dopamine and nondopamine receptors. J Neurosci 20:3504–3511, 2000

Shimosato K, Tomita M, Ijiri I: Urinary excretion of p-hydroxylated methamphetamine metabolites in man, I: a method for determination by high-performance liquid chromatography-electrochemistry. Arch Toxicol 59:135–140, 1986

Shoptaw S, Heinzerling KG, Rotheram-Fuller E, et al: Randomized, placebo-controlled trial of bupropion for the treatment of methamphetamine dependence. Drug Alcohol Depend 96:222–232, 2008

Simonini MV, Polak PE, Sharp A, et al: Increasing CNS noradrenaline reduces EAE severity. J Neuroimmune Pharmacol 5:252–259, 2010

Sinnott RS, Mach RH, Nader MA: Dopamine D2/D3 receptors modulate cocaine's reinforcing and discriminative stimulus effects in rhesus monkeys. Drug Alcohol Depend 54:97–110, 1999

Skelton MR, Williams MT, Schaefer TL, et al: Neonatal (+)-methamphetamine increases brain derived neurotrophic factor, but not nerve growth factor, during treatment and results in long-term spatial learning deficits. Psychoneuroendocrinology 32:734–745, 2007

Smythies J: Section III. The norepinephrine system. Int Rev Neurobiol 64:173–211, 2005

Snyder SH, Coyle JT: Regional differences in H3-norepinephrine and H3-dopamine uptake into rat brain homogenates. J Psychopharmacol Exp Ther 165:78–86, 1969

Sofuoglu M: Cognitive enhancement as a pharmacotherapy target for stimulant addiction. Addiction 105:38–48, 2010

Sofuoglu M, Sewell RA: Norepinephrine and stimulant addiction. Addict Biol 14:119–129, 2009

Sofuoglu M, Poling J, Waters A, et al: Disulfiram enhances subjective effects of dextroamphetamine in humans. Pharmacol Biochem Behav 90:394–398, 2008

Sofuoglu M, Poling J, Hill K, et al: Atomoxetine attenuates dextroamphetamine effects in humans. Am J Drug Alcohol Abuse 35:412–416, 2009

Sofuoglu M, Mooney M, Kosten T, et al: Minocycline attenuates subjective rewarding effects of dextroamphetamine in humans. Psychopharmacology (Berl) 213:61–68, 2011

Solinas M, Panlilio LV, Justinova Z, et al: Using drug-discrimination techniques to study the abuse-related effects of psychoactive drugs in rats. Nat Protoc 1:1194–1206, 2006

Sonsalla PK, Nicklas WJ, Heikkila RE: Role for excitatory amino acids in methamphetamine-induced nigrostriatal dopaminergic toxicity. Science 243:398–400, 1989

Sonsalla PK, Riordan DE, Heikkila RE: Competitive and noncompetitive antagonists at N-methyl-D-aspartate receptors protect against methamphetamine-induced dopaminergic damage in mice. J Psychopharmacol Exp Ther 256:506–512, 1991

Spyraki C, Fibiger HC, Phillips AG: Cocaine-induced place preference conditioning: lack of effects of neuroleptics and 6-hydroxydopamine lesions. Brain Res 253:195–203, 1982

Sriram K, Miller DB, O'Callaghan JP: Minocycline attenuates microglial activation but fails to mitigate striatal dopaminergic neurotoxicity: role of tumor necrosis factor-alpha. J Neurochem 96:706–718, 2006

Srisurapanont M, Ali R, Marsden J, et al: Psychotic symptoms in methamphetamine psychotic in-patients. Int J Neuropsychopharmacol 6:347–352, 2003

Stefanini E, Frau M, Garau MG, et al: Alcohol-preferring rats have fewer dopamine D2 receptors in the limbic system. Alcohol Alcohol 27:127–130, 1992

Stefanski R, Ladenheim B, Lee SH, et al: Neuroadaptations in the dopaminergic system after active self-administration but not after passive administration of methamphetamine. Eur J Pharmacol 371:123–135, 1999

Stefanski R, Lee SH, Yasar S, et al: Lack of persistent changes in the dopaminergic system of rats withdrawn from methamphetamine self-administration. Eur J Pharmacol 439:59–68, 2002

Stewart J, de Wit H, Eikelboom R: Role of unconditioned and conditioned drug effects in the self-administration of opiates and stimulants. Psychol Rev 91:251–268, 1984

Stoops WW, Lile JA, Glaser PE, et al: Intranasal cocaine functions as reinforcer on a progressive ratio schedule in humans. Eur J Pharmacol 644:101–105, 2010

Substance Abuse and Mental Health Services Administration: Treatment Episode Data Set (TEDS): 1998–2008. National Admissions to Substance Abuse Treatment Services (Office of Applied Studies, DASIS Series S-50, HHS Publ No SMA-09-4471). 2010. Available at: http://wwwdasis.samhsa.gov/teds08/teds2k8natweb.pdf. Accessed March 17, 2011.

Sulzer D, Sonders MS, Poulsen NW, et al: Mechanisms of neurotransmitter release by amphetamines: a review. Prog Neurobiol 75:406–433, 2005

Suzuki H, Sugimura Y, Iwama S, et al: Minocycline prevents osmotic demyelination syndrome by inhibiting the activation of microglia. J Am Soc Nephrol 21:2090–2098, 2010

Swanson LW, Hartman BK: The central adrenergic system. An immunofluorescence study of the location of cell bodies and their efferent connections in the rat utilizing dopamine-beta-hydroxylase as a marker. J Comp Neurol 163:467–505, 1975

Swant J, Chirwa S, Stanwood G, et al: Methamphetamine reduces LTP and increases baseline synaptic transmission in the CA1 region of mouse hippocampus. PloS One 5:e11382, 2010

Szumlinski KK, Ary AW, Lominac KD: Homers regulate drug-induced neuroplasticity: implications for addiction. Biochem Pharmacol 75:112–133, 2008

Tanibuchi Y, Shimagami M, Fukami G, et al: A case of methamphetamine use disorder treated with the antibiotic drug minocycline. Gen Hosp Psychiatry 32:559.e1-3, 2010

Terwilliger RZ, Beitner-Johnson D, Sevarino KA, et al: A general role for adaptations in G-proteins and the cyclic AMP system in mediating the chronic actions of morphine and cocaine on neuronal function. Brain Res 548:100–110, 1991

Thanos PK, Michaelides M, Benveniste H, et al: Effects of chronic oral methylphenidate on cocaine self-administration and striatal dopamine D2 receptors in rodents. Pharmacol Biochem Behav 87:426–433, 2007

Thomas DM, Walker PD, Benjamins JA, et al: Methamphetamine neurotoxicity in dopamine nerve endings of the striatum is associated with microglial activation. J Psychopharmacol Exp Ther 311:1–7, 2004

Thomas DM, Francescutti-Verbeem DM, Kuhn DM: The newly synthesized pool of dopamine determines the severity of methamphetamine-induced neurotoxicity. J Neurochem 105:605–616, 2008

Thomas MJ, Buerrier C, Bonci A, et al: Long-term depression in the nucleus accumbens: a neural correlate of behavioral sensitization to cocaine. Nat Neurosci 4:1217–1223, 2001

Thomas MJ, Kalivas PW, Shaham Y: Neuroplasticity in the mesolimbic dopamine system and cocaine addiction. Br J Pharmacol 154:327–342, 2008

Thompson HS: Hell's Angels, 3rd Edition. New York, Ballantine Books, 1967

Thomsen M, Han DD, Gu HH, et al: Lack of cocaine self-administration in mice expressing a cocaine-insensitive dopamine transporter. J Psychopharmacol Exp Ther 331:204–211, 2009

Tiihonen J, Kuoppasalmi K, Föhr J, et al: A comparison of aripiprazole, methylphenidate, and placebo for amphetamine dependence. Am J Psychiatry 164:160–162, 2007

Tokunaga M, Seneca N, Shin RM, et al: Neuroimaging and physiological evidence for involvement of glutamatergic transmission in regulation of the striatal dopaminergic system. J Neurosci 29:1887–1896, 2009

Tsai S: Increased central brain-derived neurotrophic factor activity could be a risk factor for substance abuse: implications for treatment. Med Hypotheses 68:410–414, 2007

Turner DC, Clark L, Dowson J, et al: Modafinil improves cognition and response inhibition in adult attention-deficit/hyperactivity disorder. Biol Psychiatry 55:1031–1040, 2004

Ujike H, Sato M: Clinical features of sensitization to methamphetamine observed in patients with methamphetamine dependence and psychosis. Ann N Y Acad Sci 1025:279–287, 2004

Ujike H, Onoue T, Akiyama K, et al: Effects of selective D-1 and D-2 dopamine antagonists on development of methamphetamine-induced behavioral sensitization. Psychopharmacology (Berl) 98:89–92, 1989

Uramura K, Yada T, Muroya S, et al: Methamphetamine induces cytosolic Ca2+ oscillations in the VTA dopamine neurons. Neuroreport 11:1057–1061, 2000

U.S. Department of Health and Human Services: National Survey on Drug Use and Health. 2009. Available at: http://www.oas.samhsa.gov/NSDUH/2k9NSDUH/2k9Results.htm. Accessed June 28, 2011.

U.S. Department of Health and Human Services: Drug Abuse Warning Network, 2005: Area Profiles of Drug-Related Mortality. 2005. Available at: http://dawninfo.samhsa.gov/files/me2005/dawn2k5me.htm. Accessed June 28, 2011.

Vanderschuren LJ, Everitt BJ: Drug seeking becomes compulsive after prolonged cocaine self-administration. Science 305:1017–1019, 2004

Vanderschuren LJ, Kalivas PW: Alterations in dopaminergic and glutamatergic transmission in the induction and expression of behavioral sensitization: a critical review of preclinical studies. Psychopharmacology (Berl) 151:99–120, 2000

Van Dyke C, Byck R, Barash PG, et al: Urinary excretion of immunologically reactive metabolite(s) after intranasal administration of cocaine, as followed by enzyme immunoassay. Clin Chem 23:241–244, 1977

Vassout A, Bruinink A, Krauss J, et al: Regulation of dopamine receptors by bupropion: comparison with antidepressants and CNS stimulants. J Recept Res 13:341–354, 1993

Vocci FJ, Montoya ID: Psychological treatments for stimulant misuse, comparing and contrasting those for amphetamine dependence and those for cocaine dependence. Curr Opin Psychiatry 22:263–268, 2009

Volkow ND, Fowler JS, Wolf AP, et al: Effects of chronic cocaine abuse on postsynaptic dopamine receptors. Am J Psychiatry 147:740–747, 1990

Volkow ND, Fowler JS, Wang GJ, et al: Decreased dopamine D2 receptor availability is associated with reduced frontal metabolism in cocaine abusers. Synapse 14:169–177, 1993

Volkow ND, Wang GJ, Fowler JS, et al: Decreases in dopamine receptors but not in dopamine transporters in alcoholics. Alcohol Clin Exp Res 20:1594–1598, 1996a

Volkow ND, Wang GJ, Fowler JS, et al: Relationship between psychostimulant-induced "high" and dopamine transporter occupancy. Proc Natl Acad Sci U S A 93:10388–10392, 1996b

Volkow ND, Fowler JS, Wang GJ: Imaging studies on the role of dopamine in cocaine reinforcement and addiction in humans. J Psychopharmacol 13:337–345, 1999a

Volkow ND, Wang GJ, Fowler JS, et al: Prediction of reinforcing responses to psychostimulants in humans by brain dopamine D2 receptor levels. Am J Psychiatry 156:1440–1443, 1999b

Volkow ND, Wang GJ, Fowler JS, et al: Reinforcing effects of psychostimulants in humans are associated with increases in brain dopamine and occupancy of D(2) receptors. J Psychopharmacol Exp Ther 291:409–415, 1999c

Volkow ND, Wang GJ, Fischman MW, et al: Effects of route of administration on cocaine induced dopamine transporter blockade in the human brain. Life Sci 67:1507–1515, 2000

Volkow ND, Chang L, Wang GJ, et al: Association of dopamine transporter reduction with psychomotor impairment in methamphetamine abusers. Am J Psychiatry 158:377–382, 2001a

Volkow ND, Chang L, Wang GJ, et al: Higher cortical and lower subcortical metabolism in detoxified methamphetamine abusers. Am J Psychiatry 158:383–389, 2001b

Volkow ND, Fowler JS, Logan J, et al: Effects of modafinil on dopamine and dopamine transporters in the male human brain: clinical implications. JAMA 301:1148–1154, 2009

Volkow ND, Wang GJ, Fowler JS, et al: Addiction: decreased reward sensitivity and increased expectation sensitivity conspire to overwhelm the brain's control circuit. Bioessays 32:748–755, 2010

Völlm BA, de Araujo IE, Cowen PJ, et al: Methamphetamine activates reward circuitry in drug naïve human subjects. Neuropsychopharmacology 29:1715–1722, 2004

Vosburg SK, Hart CL, Haney M, et al: Modafinil does not serve as a reinforcer in cocaine abusers. Drug Alcohol Depend 106:233–236, 2010

Wachtel SR, de Wit H: Subjective and behavioral effects of repeated d-amphetamine in humans. Behav Pharmacol 10:271–281, 1999

Wang GJ, Volkow ND, Fowler JS, et al: Dopamine D2 receptor availability in opiate-dependent subjects before and after naloxone-precipitated withdrawal. Neuropsychopharmacology 16:174–182, 1997

Wang GJ, Yang J, Volkow ND, et al: Gastric stimulation in obese subjects activates the hippocampus and other regions involved in brain reward circuitry. Proc Natl Acad Sci U S A 103:15641–15645, 2006

Ward AS, Haney M, Fischman MW, et al: Binge cocaine self-administration by humans: smoked cocaine. Behav Pharmacol 8:736–744, 1997a

Ward AS, Haney M, Fischman MW, et al: Binge cocaine self-administration in humans: intravenous cocaine. Psychopharmacology (Berl) 132:375–381, 1997b

The Washington Times: Coca kick in drinks spurs export fears. April 19, 2004. Available at: http://www.washingtontimes.com/news/2004/apr/19/20040419-093635-4754r. Accessed June 26, 2011.

Wayment H, Meiergerd SM, Schenk JO: Relationships between the catechol substrate binding site and amphetamine, cocaine, and mazindol binding sites in a kinetic model of the striatal transporter of dopamine in vitro. J Neurochem 70:1941–1949, 1998

Weinshenker D, Schroeder JP: There and back again: a tale of norepinephrine and drug addiction. Neuropsychopharmacology 32:1433–1451, 2007

Weinshenker D, Miller NS, Blizinsky K, et al: Mice with chronic norepinephrine deficiency resemble amphetamine-sensitized animals. Proc Natl Acad Sci U S A 99:13873–13877, 2002

Weinshenker D, Ferrucci M, Busceti CL, et al: Genetic or pharmacological blockade of noradrenaline synthesis enhances the neurochemical, behavioral, and neurotoxic effects of methamphetamine. J Neurochem 105:471–483, 2008

White NM: Addictive drugs as reinforcers: multiple partial actions on memory systems. Addiction 91:921–949; discussion 951–965, 1996

Whitehead RE, Ferrer JV, Javitch JA, et al: Reaction of oxidized dopamine with endogenous cysteine residues in the human dopamine transporter. J Neurochem 76:1242–1251, 2001

Wise RA: Catecholamine theories of reward: a critical review. Brain Res 152:215–247, 1978

Wise RA, Bozarth MA: A psychomotor stimulant theory of addiction. Psychol Rev 94:469–492, 1987

Wise RA, Rompre PP: Brain dopamine and reward. Annu Rev Psychol 40:191–225, 1989

Witkin JM, Savtchenko N, Mashkovsky M, et al: Behavioral, toxic, and neurochemical effects of sydnocarb, a novel psychomotor stimulant: comparisons with methamphetamine. J Pharmacol Exp Ther 288:1298–1310, 1999

Wu JC, Bell K, Najafi A, et al: Decreasing striatal 6-FDOPA uptake with increasing duration of cocaine withdrawal. Neuropsychopharmacology 17:402–409, 1997

Xie T, McCann UD, Kim S, et al: Effect of temperature on dopamine transporter function and intracellular accumulation of methamphetamine: implications for methamphetamine-induced dopaminergic neurotoxicity. J Neurosci 20:7838–7845, 2000

Yahyavi-Firouz-Abadi N, See RE: Anti-relapse medications: preclinical models for drug addiction treatment. Pharmacol Ther 124:235–247, 2009

Yamamoto BK, Moszczynska A, Gudelsky GA: Amphetamine toxicities: classical and emerging mechanisms. Ann N Y Acad Sci 1187:101–121, 2010

Yui K, Ikemoto S, Ishiguro T, et al: Studies of amphetamine or methamphetamine psychosis in Japan: relation of methamphetamine psychosis to schizophrenia. Ann N Y Acad Sci 914:1–12, 2000

Zhang L, Kitaichi K, Fujimoto Y, et al: Protective effects of minocycline on behavioral changes and neurotoxicity in mice after administration of methamphetamine. Prog Neuropsychopharmacol Biol Psychiatry 30:1381–1393, 2006

Zhang L, Shirayama Y, Iyo M, et al: Minocycline attenuates hyperlocomotion and prepulse inhibition deficits in mice after administration of the NMDA receptor antagonist dizocilpine. Neuropsychopharmacology 32:2004–2010, 2007

Zhang W, Ordway GA: The alpha2C-adrenoceptor modulates GABA release in mouse striatum. Brain Res Mol Brain Res 112:24–32, 2003

Zhang W, Klimek V, Farley JT, et al: Alpha2C adrenoceptors inhibit adenylyl cyclase in mouse striatum: potential activation by dopamine. J Psychopharmacol Exp Ther 289:1286–1292, 1999

Zhang X, Banjeree A, Banks WA, et al: N-Acetylcysteine amide protects against methamphetamine-induced oxidative stress and neurotoxicity in immortalized human brain endothelial cells. Brain Res 1275:87–95, 2009

Zhang XY, Kosten TA: Prazosin, an alpha-1 adrenergic antagonist, reduces cocaine-induced reinstatement of drug-seeking. Biol Psychiatry 57:1202–1204, 2005

Zhang XY, Kosten TA: Previous exposure to cocaine enhances cocaine self-administration in an alpha 1-adrenergic receptor dependent manner. Neuropsychopharmacology 32:638–645, 2007

Ziskin JL, Nishiyama A, Rubio M, et al: Vesicular release of glutamate from unmyelinated axons in white matter. Nat Neurosci 10:321–330, 2007

Zuccato E, Castiglioni S: Illicit drugs in the environment. Philos Transact A Math Phys Eng Sci 367:3965–3978, 2009

Zuo Y, Lin A, Chang P, et al: Development of long-term dendritic spine stability in diverse regions of cerebral cortex. Neuron 46:181–189, 2005

ILLUSTRATION CREDITS

Some of the figures included in this chapter are licensed for use under alternative or "copyleft" arrangements as described in this section. More information about the permitted use of these images is available at the source links below.

Figure 2–1. *Source:* Modified from: http://commons.wikimedia.org/wiki/File:Dopamine2.svg; http://en.wikipedia.org/wiki/File:Norepinephrine_structure_with_descriptor.svg; http://en.wikipedia.org/wiki/File:Epinephrine_structure_with_descriptor.svg; http://en.wikipedia.org/wiki/File:Kokain_-_Cocaine.svg; http://en.wikipedia.org/wiki/File:Amphetamine-2D-skeletal.svg; http://en.wikipedia.org/wiki/File:MDMA_%28simple%29.svg.

All accessed March 11, 2011. "I, the copyright holder of this work, release this work into the public domain. This applies worldwide. In some countries this may not be legally possible; if so: I grant anyone the right to use this work for any purpose, without any conditions, unless such conditions are required by law."

Figure 2–3. *Source:* Adapted from Dubuc B: "The Brain From Top to Bottom," [n.d.]. Available at: http://commons.wikimedia.org/wiki/File:Nucleus_accumbens.jpg [http://thebrain.mcgill.ca/flash/d/d_03/d_03_cr/d_03_cr_que/d_03_cr_que_1a.jpg].

Accessed March 11, 2011. This file is licensed under the Creative Commons Attribution-Share Alike 3.0 Unported license. You are free to share, to copy, distribute and transmit the work, to remix, to adapt the work, under the following conditions: Attribution: You must attribute the work in the manner specified by the author or licensor (but not in any way that suggests that they endorse you or your use of the work). Share alike: If you alter, transform, or build upon this work, you may distribute the resulting work only under the same or similar license to this one.

Figure 2–6. *Source:* Nutt et al. 2007. Available at: http://en.wikipedia.org/wiki/ File:Rational_scale_to_assess_the_harm_of_drugs_%28mean_physical_harm_ and_mean_dependence%29.svg.

Accessed March 11, 2011. "I, the copyright holder of this work, release this work into the public domain. This applies worldwide. In some countries this may not be legally possible; if so: I grant anyone the right to use this work for any purpose, without any conditions, unless such conditions are required by law."

Figure 2–7A. *Source:* Zell H: "*Erythroxylum coca.*" September 13, 2009. Available at: http://commons.wikimedia.org/wiki/File:Erythroxylum_coca_002.JPG.

Accessed April 13, 2011. Permission is granted to copy, distribute and/or modify this document under the terms of the GNU Free Documentation License, Version 1.2 or any later version published by the Free Software Foundation; with no Invariant Sections, no Front-Cover Texts, and no Back-Cover Texts. A copy of the license is included in the section entitled GNU Free Documentation License.

Figure 2–7B. *Source:* "Sigmund Freud–1922." Image from the Google-hosted LIFE Photo Archive, where it is available under the filename e45a47b1b422cca3. 1920. Available at: http://commons.wikimedia.org/wiki/ File:Sigmund_Freud_LIFE.jpg.

Accessed April 13, 2011. This work is in the public domain in the United States because it was published before January 1, 1923. The author died in 1940, so this work is also in the public domain in countries and areas where the copyright term is the author's life plus 70 years or less.

Figure 2–7C. *Source:* http://commons.wikimedia.org/wiki/ File:Cocaine_tooth_drops.png.

Accessed April 13, 2011. This image is in the public domain because its copyright has expired. This applies to the United States, Australia, the European Union and those countries with a copyright term of life of the author plus 70 years.

Figure 2–8. *Source:* U.S. Drug Enforcement Administration: "Cocaine Hydrochloride Powder." July 26, 2006. Available at: http://en.wikipedia.org/wiki/File:Cocaine-HydrochloridePowder.jpg [http://www.justice.gov/dea/photos/cocaine/ cocaine.jpg].

Accessed March 11, 2011. This image is a work of a Drug Enforcement Administration employee, taken or made during the course of an employee's official duties. As a work of the U.S. federal government, the image is in the public domain (17 U.S.C. § 101 and § 105).

Figure 2–9. *Source:* Psychonaught: "Blue Crystal Meth." April 5, 2010. Available at: http://en.wikipedia.org/wiki/File:Blue_Crystal_Meth_.jpg.

Accessed March 11, 2011. "I, the copyright holder of this work, release this work into the public domain. This applies worldwide. In some countries this may not be legally possible; if so: I grant anyone the right to use this work for any purpose, without any conditions, unless such conditions are required by law."

Chapter 3

Diagnoses, Symptoms, and Assessment

Thomas R. Kosten, M.D.

This chapter provides an overview of the diagnoses and assessment for stimulant abuse and dependence, including their definition in the *Diagnostic and Statistical Manual of Mental Disorders,* 4th Edition, Text Revision (DSM-IV-TR; American Psychiatric Association 2000). However, even when stimulant use is insufficient to meet these disorder criteria, the criteria may influence management and prognosis of co-occurring disorders, and recent evidence has demonstrated the effectiveness of very brief counseling sessions in reducing use and problems in patients who are not yet dependent on substances (Saitz 2005). Furthermore, the distinction between the diagnoses of *abuse* and *dependence* for cocaine or amphetamine (AMPH) is of limited clinical importance and is expected to be eliminated in DSM-5.

The definitions of substance abuse and dependence are based on the dependence syndrome of Griffith Edwards (Edwards and Gross 1976). Although this syndrome originally had 10 criteria, DSM-IV (American

Psychiatric Association 1994) reduced the number of criteria for dependence to seven, including tolerance and withdrawal (Criteria 1 and 2) and a pattern of compulsive use (Criteria 3 through 7). The DSM-IV criteria were retained in DSM-IV-TR. The severity of dependence can be indicated by the number of criteria met (from a minimum of three to a maximum of seven) and by whether or not physiological dependence occurs (i.e., whether there is tolerance or withdrawal), because physiological dependence is associated with a higher risk for immediate general medical problems and a higher relapse rate. The five criteria indicating compulsive use alone may define substance dependence if at least three occur at any time in the same 12-month period. Individuals with stimulant dependence tend to demonstrate a wide variability in the number of dependence criteria met, with the proportion of patients having relatively low levels of dependence approximately equal to those having extremely high levels of dependence.

Substance abuse is a maladaptive pattern of substance use leading to significant adverse consequences, manifested by psychosocial, medical, or legal problems or use in situations in which it is physically hazardous, recurring within a 12-month period. Since a diagnosis of stimulant dependence preempts a diagnosis of abuse, the three criteria of tolerance, withdrawal, and compulsive use are generally not present in individuals with a diagnosis of stimulant abuse.

When the clinician is considering a diagnosis of stimulant use disorder, obtaining accurate information about adult and, particularly, teenage drug use can be a major problem. Even when derived from anonymous or confidential reports, information about teenage drug use may include socially acceptable but untruthful answers such as simply, "I don't." In a recent prospective cohort of high-risk urban youth, the concordance between confidential self- and parent report of teen cocaine use with biomarkers (hair analysis) was poor (Delaney-Black et al. 2010). The teens' biological tests (i.e., drug analytes in hair) showed a substantially greater rate of use than was obtained by either teen self-report or parent report. In the more than 400 teens in the cohort, the hair specimens were 52 times more likely to identify cocaine use compared with self-report. Parent hair analyses for cocaine use were 6.5 times more likely to indicate drug use than was parent self-report. The lack of concordance between self-report and bioassay occurred despite participants' knowledge that a "certificate of confidentiality" protected both teen and adult participants and that the biological specimens would be tested for drugs. Urine tests for stimulants cannot be expected to yield such dramatic underreporting of use, because urine tests are only positive for about 72 hours, compared with the 3-month window of detection for hair analyses. Thus, only very recent use would be detected from urine samples. Nevertheless, some type of biological assessment for stimulant use is essential for reasonable detection through screening of high-risk groups for stimulant abuse. The SBIRT (Screening, Brief Intervention, and Referral to Treatment), a national program for screening and brief interventions with drug abusers, indicates that such urine screening in emergency departments has particularly high yields for detection and for reducing health care utilization with even a single, brief, 10- to 15-minute intervention focused on the substance abuse (Office of National Drug Control Policy 2008).

Clinical Aspects of Stimulant Use

The subjective and behavioral responses to stimulants are very complex and depend on many variables, including 1) dose, 2) route of administration (intravenous administration and smoking produce an intensely pleasurable response due to a more immediate onset of euphoria), 3) previous experience with stimulants, 4) the environment in which the drug is taken, and 5) the unique response pattern of the individual user, which may in part be genetically determined.

The preferred method of self-administering cocaine has been snorting and smoking. Amphetamines come in a variety of forms, such as pill, liquid, and powder, but are usually taken orally or intravenously and sometimes smoked. In most subjects, low doses administered orally produce a sense of relaxation, well-being, diminished fatigue, self-confidence, and mental alertness (Kosten 2002; Martin et al. 1971). Increasing of doses results in greater activation, anxiety, insomnia, and anorexia, and dose escalation is necessary to maintain reinforcing properties (Foltin et al. 2003). The mood response can vary from elation to extreme dysphoria. An antidepressant effect is seen in some depressed patients (Silberman et al. 1981), and cocaine abusers with milder depressive symptoms experience enhanced effects after cocaine administration (Sofuoglu et al. 2001; Uslaner et al. 1999). However, some studies suggest that individuals with primary depression (i.e., not substance induced) have dysphoric responses to cocaine (Rosenblum et al. 1999).

Stimulant use may range from low-dose to high-dose and from infrequent to chronic or binge patterns. Depending on the dosage, pattern, and duration of use, stimulants can produce several drug-induced states that differ in clinical characteristics. Moderate to high doses of stimulants can produce stimulant intoxication that may or may not be pleasant. The intoxicated person may show signs of hyperawareness, hypersexuality, hypervigilance, and psychomotor agitation. Often the symptoms of stimulant-induced intoxication resemble mania. The intoxicated person should be monitored by medical staff until the symptoms of intoxication diminish. If the intoxication does not return to baseline level within 24 hours, mania may be present and treatment for manic disorder may be required (Gawin and Ellinwood 1988).

With increased dosage and duration of administration, stimulants can also produce a state of mental confusion and excitement, known as stimulant delirium. Delirium is associated with becoming disoriented and confused, as well as anxious and fearful. Extreme medical caution is needed when treating delirium, because such symptoms may indicate stimulant overdose. For instance, crack cocaine addicts who overdose need careful monitoring for seizures, cardiac arrhythmias, stroke, and pulmonary complications. Overdose management has been reviewed in detail (Gay 1982), but a syndrome of hyperthermia and agitation might be most safely managed with high doses of benzodiazepines (Kosten and Kleber 1988).

Stimulants induce both tolerance and sensitization to their behavioral effects. Tolerance develops to the anorectic and euphoric effects of stimulants (Schuster 1981); however, chronic intermittent use of low doses of stimulants delays the development of tolerance. In doses commonly used in clinical practice, patients treated for narcolepsy or depressive or apathetic states find that the stimulant properties usually persist without development of tolerance; however, the persistence of antidepressant effects remains a matter of controversy. Sensitization has been linked to the development of AMPH-induced psychosis (Yui et al. 1999). Sensitization to the induction of psychosis is suggested because psychosis is induced by progressively lower doses and shorter periods of consumption of AMPH following repeated use over time (Sato 1992). Sensitization for AMPH-induced psychosis may persist despite long periods of abstinence.

During high-dose stimulant use, often seen during binge episodes, individuals can experience stimulant-induced psychosis characterized by delusions, paranoid thinking, and stereotyped compulsive behavior. When the patient is delusional, close clinical monitoring is essential, and it may be necessary to employ short-term treatment with neuroleptics to ameliorate the psychosis. It is more common for AMPH than for cocaine to induce psychosis, perhaps due to the difficulty in maintaining high chronic levels of cocaine in the body. Also, stimulant-induced psychosis in humans may be related to the dose and duration of AMPH administration, although cocaine psychosis and paranoia may be related to psychiatric predisposition (King and Ellinwood 1997). The amphetamines, methylphenidate, and phenmetrazine all produce psychosis (Ellinwood et al. 1973; Harris and Batki 2000; Iversen et al. 1978; Lucas and Weiss 1971; McCormick and McNeil 1962). Some authorities believe that psychosis is more common with binge patterns of use and escalating dosages (Gawin 1991; Segal and Kuczenski 1997). Compared with other stimulants, cocaine appears less likely to lead to psychosis, for reasons that are probably related to dose and patterns of use. Most individuals use cocaine intermittently, whereas daily use of AMPH is common (King and Ellinwood 1997). Susceptibility to stimulant-induced psychosis may also be related to differences in the effects of various stimulants on monoamines (Fleckenstein et al. 2000; Vanderschuren and Kalivas 2000). Some (Janowsky et al. 1973), but not all (Kornetsky 1976), patients with schizophrenia are sensitive to exacerbation of psychosis from stimulants. Paranoid delusions can probably be induced in most people if an adequate dose of stimulant is given (Griffith et al. 1968). Patients with schizophrenia who are cocaine dependent may have more hallucinations than patients presenting with either disorder alone, although there is considerable similarity in clinical presentations (Serper et al. 1999). The dose required to produce psychosis varies greatly among individuals (Bell 1973). It has been estimated that 50% of people who abuse AMPH at a dosage of 30–100 mg/day for 3 months will develop psychotic symptoms (Sato 1992).

Prior to the onset of overt psychosis, most stimulant users begin to exhibit suspiciousness and a fascination with details of objects in their environment and often will begin to perform repetitive behaviors, such as picking at their skin, disassembling mechanical objects, and prolonged masturbation or coitus (Connell 1958). With higher doses or continued administration, users begin to experience paranoid delusions; ideas of reference; visual, auditory, or olfactory hallucinations; and agitation (Ellinwood 1967). Violence, including homicide, has been reported as a consequence of this activated, paranoid state (Ellinwood 1967; Kramer 1969). The combination of alcohol and cocaine appears to be an especially high risk factor for violent behavior, even in the absence of psychotic symptoms (Chermack and Blow 2002). Disorientation (stimulant delirium) appears in some instances. A syndrome of hyperthermia and agitation that resembles neuroleptic malignant syndrome has also been reported (Kosten and Kleber 1988).

The clinical presentation of stimulant psychosis has frequently been described as being indistinguishable from paranoid schizophrenia (Angrist and Gershon 1970; Ellinwood 1971). Supporting the similarity is a study that examined the symptoms of psychosis in 168 methamphetamine (METH)-dependent inpatients in Australia, Japan, the Philippines, and Thailand, which found that 77% of the subjects had experienced persecutory delusions during their lifetime "followed by auditory hallucinations, strange or unusual beliefs, and thought reading" (Srisurapanont et al. 2003). Almost half of the subjects experienced auditory hallucinations, followed by strange or unusual beliefs and visual hallucinations. Twenty percent of the subjects exhibited negative symptoms (i.e., "poverty of speech, psychomotor retardation, and flattened/incongruous affects") resembling a schizophreniform disorder. Some clinical presentations may be confused with acute mania, characterized by agitation, hypersexuality, affective lability, and grandiosity.

In addition, many symptoms, such as olfactory hallucinations, déjà vu, and philosophical preoccupation, and the very atypical course of the illness are suggestive of temporal lobe epilepsy (Ellinwood 1968). Stimulant psychosis generally clears within a few days of discontinuation of the drug (Beamish and Kiloh 1960; Spear and Alderton 2003), although prolonged psychoses are sometimes associated with stimulant abuse (Ahmad 2003; Iversen et al. 1978). Stimulant psychosis is generally managed by close psychiatric and medical supervision, and judicious use of benzodiazepines and atypical antipsychotics (Jha and Fourie 1999; Misra and Kofoed 1997).

Dependence and withdrawal can occur with all stimulants. Cocaine is one of the most strongly reinforcing drugs in self-administration paradigms in animals, and it also has a psychological withdrawal syndrome. Stimulant withdrawal can produce a wide range of dysphoric symptoms. Following binge use, individuals may initially experience a "crash" period, which is characterized by symptoms of depression, anxiety, agitation, and intense drug craving, although controlled studies have shown minimal withdrawal symptoms (Gawin and Ellinwood 1988; Volkow et al. 1990). This syndrome may last for several days after the drug is withdrawn. Since tolerance develops quickly, abusers may take large doses compared with those used medically (e.g., as anorexiants).

Assessment

Because diagnosis should lead to treatment for stimulant use disorders, diagnoses require a comprehensive assessment of the patient's psychological, medical, forensic, and drug use history. Moreover, because information obtained from chemically dependent persons may be incomplete or unreliable, it is important that the patients receive a thorough physical, including blood and supervised urine samples for analysis. The clinician needs to be aware that polydrug abuse is common (see Chapter 6, this volume). Patients may ingest large amounts of one or more drugs at potentially lethal doses, and therefore it is important that the physician be aware of the dangers of possible drug combinations, such as cocaine and alcohol or heroin.

Urine toxicology is as essential as self-reports for making the diagnosis of cocaine dependence and for deciding whether the patient no longer meets the criteria for this diagnosis after treatment. The frequency of urine monitoring during treatment may be as little as weekly, but three times weekly is optimal. There appears to be no advantage to quantitative over simple qualitative results based on typical cutoffs such as 300 ng/mL of benzoylecgonine for cocaine use in routine clinical practice.

The issues of motivation for seeking treatment and a tendency to deny substance use can have important influences on the patient's presentation. The patient who presents for treatment because of dysphoric feelings in the context of drug dependence is likely to articulate the severity of his or her problem adequately and even exaggerate some aspects of present discomfort. In contrast, the truck driver forced to come to a treatment program because of a driving-while-intoxicated offense is likely to minimize AMPH use or any associated complications.

Special Issues in the Psychiatric Examination

Two special issues in the psychiatric examination of substance dependence include 1) the source of information when obtaining the history of substance use and related problems and 2) the management of aberrant behaviors. Information about a patient's substance use history can be provided not only by the patient but also by employers, family members, and school officials. When a patient self-reports the amount of substance used, there is a tendency to underreport the severity and duration of use, particularly if the patient is being referred to treatment by an outside source, such as the family, the employer, or the legal system. As indicated earlier in this chapter, even when no outside referral source is leading to underreporting, hair specimens have been found to be 52 times more likely to identify cocaine use compared with self-report from adolescents (Delaney-Black et al. 2010). Parent hair analyses for cocaine use were 6.5 times more likely to indicate drug use than was parent self-report in that study. Objective verification of the exact amount of substance use is sometimes difficult, but the critical issues in arriving at a diagnosis of substance dependence do not depend on the precise amount of substance used. In general, significant others' estimates of the amount of drug use by the patient can be a good source of data. Standardized assessment tools such as the Drug Abuse Screening Test (DAST; Yudko et al. 2007) and the Addiction Severity Index (ASI; McLellan et al. 1980) may assist in both the diagnosis and treatment planning. Thus, the initial evaluation of stimulant dependence may involve a wider range of interviews than would occur with many other types of psychiatric patients.

Aberrant behaviors of intoxication, violence, suicide, impaired cognitive functioning, and uncontrolled affective displays are relatively common in these patients and require clinical management during the assessment. The evaluation of an intoxicated patient can address only a limited number of issues related to the patient's and other individuals' safety. A medical evaluation for signs of overdose or major cognitive impairment is critical, and the patient may need to be detained for several hours or even days if severe complications are evident. When a patient drives a car to an evaluation and is obviously intoxicated, the psychiatrist has an obligation to prevent the patient from getting back into the driver's seat of that vehicle until the effects of that drug intoxication have worn off. This may involve contacting the police to restrain the patient from driving, at least temporarily. Similar issues of police restraint can arise when an intoxicated patient becomes violent and has threatened to harm his or her employers or family members. Judgment and impulse control may be substantially affected by stimulants alone or in combination with other drugs or alcohol, but these effects may be temporary, and a short-term preventive intervention may be sufficient to avert substantial harm to the patient or others.

Temporary suicidal behavior may be encountered in stimulant abusers. Suicidal ideation may be intense but may clear within hours. During the evaluation session, it is important to elicit the precipitants that led the patient to seek treatment at this time and to keep the evaluation focused on specific data needed for the evaluation of the substance dependence, its medical complications, and any comorbid psychiatric disorders. Many patients spend a great deal of time detailing their drug-abusing careers, but in general these stories do not provide useful material for the evaluation or for future psychotherapeutic interventions. Similarly, the evaluation should not become focused on the affective aspects of a patient's recent life, because affect is frequently used as a defense to avoid discussing issues of more immediate relevance, such as precipitants, or used as a pretext for obtaining benzodiazepines or other anti-anxiety agents from the physician. Stimulants have generally been a way of managing and producing strong affects, and these patients need to develop alternative coping strategies.

Associated Laboratory Findings

Laboratory analyses of blood and urine samples can help determine recent use of a stimulant. Blood concentrations offer additional information on the amount of stimulant still present in the body. It should be noted 1) that a positive blood or urine test does not by itself indicate the individual has a pattern of stimulant use meeting criteria for a stimulant-related disorder, and 2) that a negative blood or urine test does not by itself rule out such a diagnosis.

In the case of intoxication, blood and urine tests can help to determine the relevant stimulant(s) involved. Specific confirmation of the suspected stimulant may require toxicological analysis, because various stimulants have similar intoxication syndromes, and individuals often take a number of different substances. Also, because substitution and contamination of street drugs are frequent, those who obtain substances illicitly often do not know the specific contents of what they have taken. Toxicological tests may also be helpful in differential diagnosis to determine the role of stimulant intoxication or withdrawal in the etiology (or exacerbation) of symptoms of a variety of mental disorders (e.g., mood disorders, psychotic disorders as described below in the section "Associated Physical Examination Findings and Psychiatric Conditions"). Furthermore, serial blood levels may help to differentiate intoxication from withdrawal.

The blood concentration of a stimulant may be a useful clue in determining whether the person has a high tolerance to it. Assessing tolerance by determining the individual's response to an agonist medication has some utility for sedatives, but this approach is not used for stimulants, since stimulant tolerance resolves within a few days and further stimulant administration in a patient who recently took them can be medically dangerous. Furthermore, there is no medical need for treatment to prevent the development of stimulant withdrawal.

Laboratory tests can be useful in identifying withdrawal from another drug that is masked or exacerbated by concurrent stimulant dependence. Evidence for cessation or reduction of dosing may be obtained by history or by toxicological analysis of body fluids (e.g., urine or blood). Most stimulants and their metabolites clear the urine within 48–72 hours after ingestion, although individuals who use stimulants daily and heavily may show these metabolites for a longer period. If the person presents with withdrawal from an unknown substance, urine tests may help identify both the substance from which the person is withdrawing and any concurrent stimulant intoxication, which can exacerbate sedative and alcohol withdrawal symptoms. Overall, these metabolite data can make it possible to initiate appropriate treatment. Urine tests may also be helpful in differentiating between withdrawal and other mental disorders, because withdrawal symptoms can mimic the symptoms of mental disorders unrelated to use of a stimulant.

Associated Physical Examination Findings and Psychiatric Conditions

Intoxication and withdrawal states are likely to include physical signs and symptoms that are often the first clue to a substance-related state. In general, intoxication with amphetamines or cocaine is accompanied by increases in blood pressure, respiratory rate, pulse, and body temperature. This set of findings contrasts with intoxication from sedative, hypnotic, or anxiolytic substances or with opioid medications, which typically involve the opposite pattern. Stimulant use disorders are often associated with general medical conditions that are related to the toxic effects of the substances on particular organ systems or to the routes of administration (e.g., nasal septum erosion due to snorting cocaine). Stimulant-related disorders are also commonly co-morbid with, and complicate the course and treatment of, many mental disorders (e.g., conduct disorder in adolescents; antisocial and borderline personality disorders, schizophrenia, bipolar disorder). An additional diagnosis of a stimulant-induced disorder is usually not made when symptoms of preexisting mental disorders are exacerbated by stimulant intoxication or stimulant withdrawal (although a diagnosis of stimulant intoxication or withdrawal might be appropriate).

Differences in Developmental, Gender, and Cultural Presentations

The most important impact of stimulant abuse or dependence during adolescence, in addition to disrupted schooling, is its direct hormonal effects. For example, stimulants can increase corticosteroid and testosterone levels. These hormonal effects can have a direct impact on the expression of secondary sex characteristics as well as sexual behaviors during adolescence. Another critical developmental effect is during the gestational period of unborn children of substance-using mothers. These children may be born with behavioral abnormalities secondary to the substance misuse by their mothers—for example, the hyperactivity that has been noted in infants born to cocaine-dependent mothers.

Sex differences in the presentation of stimulant addiction problems can be related to the setting in which these problems are detected. For example, young women may come to the attention of the substance abuse treatment provider during or soon after pregnancy, when a meconium sample detects stimulants in a premature infant. Some drug abuse patterns are also more common in women than in men. For example, the phenomenon of sex for crack frequently occurs in female cocaine addiction, but men infrequently obtain cocaine using this approach. In general, the criminal justice system is more likely to identify substance addiction in males and to insist that they get ongoing treatment as a condition of parole or probation.

Cultural differences in the presentation of stimulant use can be striking. For example, the native inhabitants of Peru use cocaine orally to adjust to their high-altitude environment and show little evidence for abuse. As another example, truckers who use AMPH to allow them to remain awake for long drives are quite different from the METH abusers in rural America. However, the relative lack of information about cultural differences in stimulant use among adolescents has led to large empirical studies such as the Monitoring the Future project. This survey has examined the prevalence, trends, and sociodemographic correlates of drug use among nationally representative samples of eighth, tenth, and twelfth graders since 1975. By twelfth grade, African American youth have the lowest use of stimulants, white youth the middle level of use, and Hispanic youth report the most stimulant use (Johnston et al. 2010).

Course and Natural History

The natural history of stimulant dependence characteristically follows the course of a chronic relapsing disorder, although a large number of individuals who experiment with stimulants in adolescence do not go on to acquire dependence. The initial phase of the natural history of experimenting with drugs has been well described in studies by Kandel (1975), who has used the concept of gateway drug use and its evolution into more serious drug dependence during adolescence and the early 20s. The later phases of dependence were characterized in the 20- to 30-year follow-up studies of individuals with alcoholism and those with opioid addiction by Vaillant, but the equivalent studies do not yet exist for stimulants (Laub and Vaillant 2000; Vaillant 1983, 1988). He has documented the natural history after age 20 years in delinquent boys (which is most closely synonymous with having lifetime conduct disorder using DSM-IV criteria) and found high mortality rates by age 40 years in those delinquent boys who later became substance users. In his most recent studies following 475 delinquent boys and 456 matched nondelinquent comparison boys from age 14 years to age 65 years, Vaillant found that 13% of the delinquent and only 6% ($n=28$) of the nondelinquent subjects died unnatural deaths. These deaths were significantly associated with abuse of alcohol during adulthood and childhood delinquency, and these two factors completely accounted for the other associations with the increased mortality, including adult crime, dysfunctional home environment, and poor education. Thus, using substances may have a critical impact on later health, but having a conduct disorder as a child increases this risk, perhaps due to related behaviors such as unwillingness to seek out appropriate

health care. Clearly, similar studies about stimulant abuse and childhood behaviors would be most informative and are now possible, as the adolescents
who started stimulants in the early 1980s would now be almost 50 years old.

The course of substance dependence is variable and may involve full or partial remission; six course specifiers are available in DSM-IV. A patient with dependence is considered to be "in remission" when none of the dependence or
abuse criteria are met for at least 1 month. Remission can then be further characterized as either early (less than 12 months) or sustained (lasting 12 months
or longer), and partial (one or more criteria for abuse or dependence are met) or
full (no criteria for dependence or abuse are met). Because the first year of remission carries a particularly high risk for relapse, it has been chosen as the
minimum required time for sustained remission. Two additional specifiers apply for special circumstances, such as when the patient is receiving agonist therapy or is in a controlled environment (e.g., jail or a therapeutic community),
where access to substances is potentially limited.

Outcome studies across substance type and treatment setting consistently show decreases in substance use, associated problems, and societal
costs. Among treated patients, 40%–60% will enter full remission, with an
additional 15%–30% achieving partial remission. The most substantial cost
benefits come from reduced crime, increased productivity, and decreased
health care costs (McLellan et al. 2000).

Differential Diagnosis

The differential diagnosis of stimulant-induced intoxication and withdrawal
can involve a wide range of psychiatric disorders. Distinguishing intoxication and withdrawal from these other disorders is usually facilitated by a
structured interview to elicit whether the range of psychiatric symptoms is
appropriately timed after the most recent stimulant use. During acute intoxication in polydrug users, the differential diagnosis might include an acute
psychotic disorder, mania, delirium, dementia, and several specific anxiety
disorders. Among these anxiety disorders are generalized anxiety disorder,
panic disorder, and obsessive-compulsive disorder. Distinguishing these disorders from acute intoxication or withdrawal with a mixture of drugs most
frequently requires that the psychiatrist wait 24–72 hours to determine
whether the symptoms persist and, therefore, whether they are independent
of the drug use. While the DSM-IV criteria for substance-induced disorders
suggest waiting for a "substantial period of time" (e.g., about a month) to
distinguish various substance-induced disorders from those not related to
substance abuse, the introduction of pharmacological treatments, such as

antidepressants, does not require such a lengthy delay. Thus, diagnostic and therapeutic distinctions may require different time frames for making clinical decisions when evaluating the patient.

A previous history of schizophrenia, bipolar disorder, or other major psychiatric disorder that is consistent with the presenting symptoms may also be helpful in arriving at an accurate diagnosis. When patients present with psychotic or manic behavior during drug intoxication, it may be necessary to use symptomatic treatment, such as with a benzodiazepine or neuroleptic agent, to conduct an examination. Because neuroleptic agents lower the seizure threshold, they are most often used in conjunction with a benzodiazepine or other anticonvulsant. A symptomatic response to neuroleptics should not be considered confirmation of an underlying diagnosis of psychotic disorder, however.

Antisocial and borderline personality disorders are commonly considered in the differential diagnosis of stimulant-dependent patients. Many of the behaviors that characterize these personality disorders are also common to the use of illegal and illicit drugs. In establishing these personality disorders, particularly antisocial personality, it is important to ascertain whether the behaviors are independent of the activities needed to obtain drugs. If many of the antisocial or borderline characteristics are specifically tied to the patient's use of drugs, these characteristics should resolve with drug abstinence and should not be considered diagnostic of a personality disorder.

The symptoms of stimulant withdrawal frequently overlap with those of depressive disorders, and this differential diagnosis can be particularly difficult. Furthermore, the syndrome of protracted withdrawal can include sleep and appetite disturbance as well as dysphoria that mimics dysthymic disorder and other affective disorders. With stimulants, depressive symptoms may persist after acute detoxification, which leads to a more difficult differential diagnosis. Thus, conservatively, the psychiatrist should wait 4–6 weeks after acute detoxification to determine a diagnosis of affective disorder in these stimulant-dependent patients. However, waiting this long is often impractical in the clinical setting, where the maintenance of sustained abstinence may depend on relief of depressive symptoms using either medications or psychotherapy. In this regard, clinical compromises are frequently needed for appropriate care in an outpatient setting.

Clinical Vignette

A 32-year-old man who had abused METH from age 18 to 21 was currently in remission but now presented with major depressive disorder. Because his depression had been refractory to selective serotonin reuptake inhibitors, monoamine oxidase inhibitors, tricyclic antidepressants, and augmentation using lithium or thyroid hormone, methylphenidate was added to maintenance treatment with a tricyclic antidepressant. The psychiatrist warned the patient about the risk in prescribing methylphenidate, given his past problems with METH, and warned that a medication change might be necessary if he experienced a stimulant-like high from the methylphenidate. Within 3 weeks, the patient called the psychiatrist, telling him that he had been taking twice the daily prescribed number of pills. The psychiatrist recognized a developing addiction to methylphenidate and began to taper the schedule of methylphenidate administration. Within 3 days, the patient had exhausted a week's supply. The psychiatrist then informed the patient that outpatient detoxification had failed and recommended hospitalization.

This case illustrates how a psychiatrist is often confronted with the issue of whether to use an addictive medication to treat a primary psychiatric disorder in a patient who also has a known substance use disorder. This dilemma is common in assessments of substance abusers in remission. Should a patient with stimulant dependence in remission with a certain diagnosis of residual attention-deficit disorder be given a trial of methylphenidate?

This clinical question often arises: Is use of addictive medications flatly contraindicated in patients with substance dependence in remission, or is such medication prohibited only in instances of use of drugs of the same class (e.g., methylphenidate and METH or cocaine)? In general, a psychiatrist should never rule out the use of any addictive drug if there are good symptom-based reasons for prescribing it. Nor should the psychiatrist assume that an addicting drug of one class (e.g., opiates) will be safe for an individual who abused another class, such as stimulants. However, in any situation in which a potentially addicting drug is considered for use in a remitted substance user, considerable caution and limit setting are warranted. Finally, inpatient management may become necessary for the evaluation and use of these risky treatment interventions.

Biomarkers for Stimulant Dependence: Future Developments

Biomarkers for stimulant and particularly cocaine dependence include abnormalities in neurotransmitter receptors and transporters, which have been noted in animal models and confirmed in human neuroimaging studies of both the dopamine (DA) and serotonin (5-HT) neurotransmitter systems (Malison et al. 1998; Sevarino et al. 2000; Volkow et al. 1990, 1992, 1996a). Single-photon emission computed tomography and positron emission tomography show increases in the dopamine transporter (DAT) during acute cocaine abstinence relative to control subjects (Malison et al. 1998), decreases in DA D_2 receptor binding in detoxified cocaine abusers (Volkow et al. 1996b), and reduced cerebral blood flow (rCBF) among chronic cocaine users (Holman et al. 1991; Kosten et al. 1998). During abstinence, this rCBF was found to improve in cocaine-dependent individuals, suggesting that drug-induced alterations may be reversed to some extent (Holman et al. 1993; Kosten 1998). Alterations in glucose metabolism have also been observed with chronic and acute stimulant administration. During early withdrawal, there was an increase in glucose metabolism among cocaine users relative to control subjects, but during late withdrawal, metabolic activity was decreased among cocaine addicts (Volkow et al. 1996a, 1992). Such reductions in glucose metabolism have also been observed following acute administration of cocaine (London et al. 1990). Most recently, decreased gray matter concentration has been described in a variety of cortical areas, including the frontal, cingulate, and temporal regions (Franklin et al. 2002).

Neuroendocrine challenge studies show functional defects consistent with these neuroimaging findings, and norepinephrine (NE) systems that stimulants might also disrupt show parallel pharmacological challenge abnormalities, such as lowered thresholds for yohimbine induction of panic attacks (Aronson et al. 1995; Bowers et al. 1998; McDougle et al. 1992, 1994; Swartz et al. 1990). These three neurotransmitter systems—DA, 5-HT, and NE—show the direct actions of chronic stimulants, but other neurotransmitter systems, including the glutamate, γ-aminobutyric acid (GABA), and kappa opioid systems, are indirectly affected (Johanson and Fischman 1989; Koob 1992).

The disturbed brain structure and function following stimulant use may be the substrate for the cognitive deficits frequently described in these patients. Impairments in verbal learning, memory, and attention have been well documented in cocaine-abusing individuals (Beatty et al. 1995; Bolla et al. 1998; Di Sclafani et al. 2002; Gottschalk et al. 2001) and are correlated with reductions in blood flow among cocaine users (Woods et al. 1991). DAT reduction also appears to correlate with psychomotor impairment in METH abusers (Volkow et al. 2001).

Thus, neurochemical and physiological alterations from chronic stimulants may lead to cognitive impairments. Abnormalities in any of these systems might be appropriate biomarkers for a diagnosis of cocaine or other stimulant dependence, and more importantly, they can be biological targets to assess whether treatment has been effective in normalizing the underlying pathophysiology of this disease. We hope that the future will allow more general clinical use of these markers for diagnosis and treatment planning and monitoring, but they are unlikely to be included in DSM-5 or treatment guidelines in the next 5 years.

KEY CLINICAL CONCEPTS

- Stimulant abuse and dependence as diagnostic distinctions will be eliminated in DSM-5, but the presence of three of the seven dependence syndrome criteria will remain as the threshold for a diagnosis of dependence, and tolerance and withdrawal will be included as two of the total seven criteria.

- Severity of stimulant dependence is reasonably assessed by simply adding up the total number of dependence criteria met, with a severity of 3 to 7.

- Stimulant abuse is substantially underreported, particularly by adolescents, whose hair samples analyzed for cocaine have shown over 50 times higher rates of abuse compared with self-reported use. Thus, urine toxicology is required for any assessment of suspected stimulant abusers.

- Stimulant-induced psychosis and suicidality can be severe but typically resolve within several days.

- Special issues in assessment include management of intoxication, violence, suicidality, impaired cognitive functioning, and uncontrolled affective displays.

- Many biomarkers are being considered for future diagnostic use, including neuroimaging and neuroendocrine tests, for matching patients to appropriate medication treatments.

Resources

Galanter M, Kleber HD (eds): The American Psychiatric Publishing Textbook of Substance Abuse Treatment, 4th Edition. Washington, DC, American Psychiatric Publishing, 2008

Substance Abuse and Mental Health Services Administration: Results from the 2009 National Survey on Drug Use and Health, Vol I: Summary of National Findings (Office of Applied Studies, NSDUH Series H-38A, HHS Publ No SMA 10-4586). 2010b. Available at: http://www.oas.samhsa.gov/NSDUH/2k9NSDUH/2k9ResultsP.pdf. Accessed March 15, 2011.

References

Ahmad K: Asia grapples with spreading amphetamine abuse. Lancet 361:1878–1879, 2003

American Psychiatric Association: Diagnostic and Statistical Manual of Mental Disorders, 4th Edition. Washington, DC, American Psychiatric Association, 1994

American Psychiatric Association: Diagnostic and Statistical Manual of Mental Disorders, 4th Edition, Text Revision. Washington, DC, American Psychiatric Association, 2000

Aronson SC, Black JE, McDougle CJ, et al: Serotonergic mechanisms of cocaine effects in humans. Psychopharmacology (Berl) 119:179–185, 1995

Beamish P, Kiloh LG: Psychoses due to amphetamine consumption. J Ment Sci 106:337–343, 1960

Beatty WW, Katzung VM, Moreland VJ, et al: Neuropsychological performance of recently abstinent alcoholics and cocaine abusers. Drug Alcohol Depend 37:247–253, 1995

Bell DS: The experimental reproduction of amphetamine psychosis. Arch Gen Psychiatry 29:35–40, 1973

Bernstein E, Bernstein J, Feldman J, et al: An evidence-based alcohol screening, brief intervention and referral to treatment (SBIRT) curriculum for emergency department (ED) providers improves skills and utilization. Academic ED SBIRT Research Collaborative. Subst Abus 28(4):79–92, 2007

Bolla KI, Cadet JL, London ED: The neuropsychiatry of chronic cocaine abuse. J Neuropsychiatry Clin Neurosci 10:280–289, 1998

Bowers MB Jr, Malison RT, Seibyl JP, et al: Plasma homovanillic acid and the dopamine transporter during cocaine withdrawal. Biol Psychiatry 43:278–281, 1998

Chermack ST, Blow FC: Violence among individuals in substance abuse treatment: the role of alcohol and cocaine consumption. Drug Alcohol Depend 66:29–37, 2002

Connell PH: Amphetamine Psychosis (Maudsley Monographs No 5). London, Oxford University Press, 1958

Delaney-Black V, Chiodo LM, Hannigan JH, et al: Just say "I don't": lack of concordance between teen report and biological measures of drug use. Pediatrics 126: 887–893, 2010

Di Sclafani V, Tolou-Shams M, Price LJ, et al: Neuropsychological performance of individuals dependent on crack-cocaine, or crack-cocaine and alcohol, at 6 weeks and 6 months of abstinence. Drug Alcohol Depend 66:161–171, 2002

Edwards G, Gross MM: Alcohol dependence: provisional description of a clinical syndrome. Br Med J 1:1058–1060, 1976

Ellinwood EH Jr: Amphetamine psychosis; I: description of the individuals and process. J Nerv Ment Dis 144:273–283, 1967

Ellinwood EH Jr: Amphetamine psychosis; II: theoretical implications. Int J Neuropsychiatry 4:45–54, 1968

Ellinwood EH Jr: Assault and homicide associated with amphetamine abuse. Am J Psychiatry 127:1170–1175, 1971

Ellinwood EH Jr, Sudilovsky A, Nelson LM: Evolving behavior in the clinical and experimental amphetamine (model) psychosis. Am J Psychiatry 130:1088–1093, 1973

Fleckenstein AE, Gibb JW, Hanson GR: Differential effects of stimulants on monoaminergic transporters: pharmacological consequences and implications for neurotoxicity. Eur J Pharmacol 406:1–13, 2000

Foltin RW, Ward AS, Haney M, et al: The effects of escalating doses of smoked cocaine
in humans. Drug Alcohol Depend 70:149–157, 2003

Franklin TR, Acton PD, Maldjian JA, et al: Decreased gray matter concentration in the
insular, orbitofrontal, cingulate, and temporal cortices of cocaine patients. Biol
Psychiatry 51:134–142, 2002

Gawin FH: Cocaine addiction: psychology and neurophysiology. Science 251:1580–
1586, 1991

Gawin FH, Ellinwood EH Jr: Cocaine and other stimulants: actions, abuse and treatment. N Engl J Med 318:1173–1182, 1988

Gay GR: Clinical management of acute and chronic cocaine poisoning. Ann Emerg
Med 11:562–572, 1982

Gottschalk C, Beauvais J, Hart R, et al: Cognitive function and cerebral perfusion during cocaine abstinence. Am J Psychiatry 158:540–545, 2001

Griffith JD, Oates JA, Cavanaugh JH: Paranoid episodes induced by drug. JAMA
205:39, 1968

Harris D, Batki SL: Stimulant psychosis: symptom profile and acute clinical course.
Am J Addict 9:28–37, 2000

Holman BL, Carvalho PA, Mendelson J, et al: Brain perfusion is abnormal in cocaine-
dependent polydrug users: a study using technetium-99m-HMPAO and
ASPECT. J Nucl Med 32:1206–1210, 1991

Holman BL, Mendelson J, Garada B, et al: Regional cerebral blood flow improves with
treatment in chronic cocaine polydrug users. J Nucl Med 34:723–727, 1993

Iversen LL, Iversen SD, Snyder SH (eds): Handbook of Psychopharmacology, Vol
11: Stimulants. New York, Plenum, 1978

Janowsky DS, el-Yousel MK, Davis JM, et al: Provocation of schizophrenic symptoms
by intravenous administration of methylphenidate. Arch Gen Psychiatry
28:185–191, 1973

Jha A, Fourie H: Risperidone treatment of amphetamine psychosis (letter). Br J Psychiatry 174:366, 1999

Johanson CE, Fischman MW: The pharmacology of cocaine related to its abuse. Pharmacol Rev 41:3–52, 1989

Johnston L, O'Malley P, Bachman J, et al: Monitoring the Future: National Survey Results on Drug Use, 1975–2009, Vol I: Secondary School Students (NIH Publ No
10-7584). Bethesda, MD, National Institute on Drug Abuse, 2010

Kandel DB: Stages in adolescent involvement in drug use. Science 190:912–914, 1975

King GR, Ellinwood EH Jr: Amphetamines and other stimulants, in Substance Abuse:
A Comprehensive Textbook, 3rd Edition. Edited by Lowinson JH, Ruiz P, Mill-
man RB, et al. Maryland, MD, Williams & Wilkins, 1997, pp 207–233

Koob GF: Neural mechanisms of drug reinforcement. Ann N Y Acad Sci 654:171–
191, 1992

Kornetsky C: Hyporesponsivity of chronic schizophrenic patients to dextroamphetamine. Arch Gen Psychiatry 33:1425–1428, 1976

Kosten TR: Pharmacotherapy of cerebral ischemia in cocaine dependence. Drug Alcohol Depend 49:133–144, 1998

Kosten TR: Pathophysiology and treatment of cocaine dependence, in Neuropsychopharmacology: The Fifth Generation of Progress. Edited by Davis KL, Charney D, Coyle JT, et al. Baltimore, MD, Lippincott Williams & Wilkins, 2002, pp 1461–1473

Kosten TR, Kleber HD: Rapid death during cocaine abuse: a variant of the neuroleptic malignant syndrome? Am J Drug Alcohol Abuse 14:335–346, 1988

Kosten TR, Cheeves C, Palumbo J, et al: Regional cerebral blood flow during acute and chronic abstinence from combined cocaine-alcohol abuse. Drug Alcohol Depend 50:187–195, 1998

Kramer JC: Introduction to amphetamine abuse. J Psychedelic Drugs 2:1–16, 1969

Laub JH, Vaillant GE: Delinquency and mortality: a 50-year follow-up study of 1,000 delinquent and nondelinquent boys. Am J Psychiatry 157:96–102, 2000

London ED, Cascella NG, Wong DF, et al: Cocaine-induced reduction of glucose utilization in human brain. A study using positron emission tomography and [fluorine 18]-fluorodeoxyglucose. Arch Gen Psychiatry 47:567–574, 1990

Lucas AR, Weiss M: Methylphenidate hallucinosis. JAMA 217:1079–1081, 1971

Malison RT, Best SE, van Dyck CH, et al: Elevated striatal dopamine transporters during acute cocaine abstinence as measured by [123I] beta-CIT SPECT. Am J Psychiatry 155:832–834, 1998

Martin WR, Sloan JW, Sapira JD, et al: Physiologic, subjective, and behavioral effects of amphetamine, methamphetamine, ephedrine, phenmetrazine, and methylphenidate in man. Clin Pharmacol Ther 12:245–258, 1971

McCormick TC Jr, McNeil TW: Acute psychosis and Ritalin abuse. Tex State J Med 59:99–100, 1962

McDougle CJ, Price LH, Palumbo JM, et al: Dopaminergic responsivity during cocaine abstinence: a pilot study. Psychiatry Res 43:77–85, 1992

McDougle CJ, Black JE, Malison RT, et al: Noradrenergic dysregulation during discontinuation of cocaine use in addicts. Arch Gen Psychiatry 51:713–719, 1994

McLellan AT, Luborsky L, O'Brien CP, et al: An improved diagnostic instrument for substance abuse patients: the Addiction Severity Index. J Nerv Ment Dis 168:26–33, 1980

McLellan AT, Lewis DC, O'Brien CP, et al: Drug dependence, a chronic medical illness: implications for treatment, insurance and outcomes evaluation. JAMA 284:1689–1695, 2000

Misra L, Kofoed L: Risperidone treatment of methamphetamine psychosis (letter). Am J Psychiatry 154:1170, 1997

Office of National Drug Control Policy: Screening, Brief Intervention, Referral and Treatment. 2008. Available at: http://www.whitehousedrugpolicy.gov/treat/screen_brief_intv.html. Accessed July 8, 2011.

Rosenblum A, Fallon B, Magura S, et al: The autonomy of mood disorders among cocaine-using methadone patients. Am J Drug Alcohol Abuse 25:67–80, 1999

Saitz R: Clinical practice: unhealthy alcohol use. N Engl J Med 352:596–607, 2005

Sato M: A lasting vulnerability to psychosis in patients with previous methamphetamine psychosis. Ann N Y Acad Sci 654:160–170, 1992

Schuster CR: The behavioral pharmacology of psychomotor stimulant drugs, in Psychotropic Agents, Part 11. Edited by Hoffmeister F, Still G. New York, Springer-Verlag, 1981, pp 587–605

Segal DS, Kuczenski R: Behavioral alterations induced by an escalating dose-binge pattern of cocaine administration. Behav Brain Res 88:251–260, 1997

Serper MR, Chou JC, Allen MH, et al: Symptomatic overlap of cocaine intoxication and acute schizophrenia at emergency presentation. Schizophr Bull 25:387–394, 1999

Sevarino KA, Oliveto A, Kosten TR: Neurobiological adaptations to psychostimulants and opiates as a basis of treatment development. Ann N Y Acad Sci 909:51–87, 2000

Silberman EK, Reus VI, Jimerson DC, et al: Heterogeneity of amphetamine response in depressed patients. Am J Psychiatry 138:1302–1307, 1981

Sofuoglu M, Brown S, Babb DA, et al: Depressive symptoms modulate the subjective and physiological response to cocaine in humans. Drug Alcohol Depend 63:131–137, 2001

Spear J, Alderton D: Psychosis associated with prescribed dexamphetamine use (letter). Aust N Z J Psychiatry 37:383, 2003

Srisurapanont M, Ali R, Marsden J, et al: Psychotic symptoms in methamphetamine psychotic in-patients. Int J Neuropsychopharmacol 6:347–352, 2003

Swartz CM, Breen K, Leone F: Serum prolactin levels during extended cocaine abstinence. Am J Psychiatry 147:777–779, 1990

Uslaner J, Kalechstein A, Richter T, et al: Association of depressive symptoms during abstinence with the subjective high produced by cocaine. Am J Psychiatry 156:1444–1446, 1999

Vaillant GE: Natural History of Alcoholism. Cambridge, MA, Harvard University Press, 1983

Vaillant GE: What can long-term follow-up teach us about relapse and prevention of relapse in addiction? Br J Addict 83:1147–1157, 1988

Vanderschuren LJ, Kalivas PW: Alterations in dopaminergic and glutamatergic transmission in the induction and expression of behavioral sensitization: a critical review of preclinical studies. Psychopharmacology (Berl) 15:99–120, 2000

Volkow ND, Fowler JS, Wolf AP, et al: Effects of chronic cocaine abuse on postsynaptic dopamine receptors. Am J Psychiatry 147:719–724, 1990

Volkow ND, Hitzemann R, Wang GJ, et al: Long-term frontal brain metabolic changes in cocaine abusers. Synapse 11:184–190, 1992

Volkow ND, Ding YS, Fowler JS, et al: Cocaine addiction: hypothesis derived from imaging studies with PET. J Addict Dis 15:55–71, 1996a

Volkow ND, Fowler JS, Gatley SJ, et al: PET evaluation of the dopamine system of the human brain. J Nucl Med 37:1242–1256, 1996b

Volkow ND, Chang L, Wang GJ, et al: Association of dopamine transporter reduction with psychomotor impairment in methamphetamine abusers. Am J Psychiatry 158:377–382, 2001

Woods SW, O'Malley SS, Martini BL, et al: SPECT regional cerebral blood flow and neuropsychological testing in non-demented HIV-positive drug abusers: preliminary results. Prog Neuropsychopharmacol Biol Psychiatry 15:649–662, 1991

Yudko E, Lozhkina O, Fouts A: A comprehensive review of the psychometric properties of the Drug Abuse Screening Test. J Subst Abuse Treat 32:189–198, 2007

Yui K, Goto K, Ikemoto S, et al: Neurobiological basis of relapse prediction in stimulant-induced psychosis and schizophrenia: the role of sensitization. Mol Psychiatry 4:512–523, 1999

Chapter 4

Behavioral Interventions

Jin H. Yoon, Ph.D.
Rachel Fintzy, M.A.
Carrie L. Dodrill, Ph.D.

A variety of behavioral interventions, either as stand-alone treatments or in conjunction with other pharmacological or behavioral-based interventions, are efficacious in addressing stimulant dependence. Behavioral treatments are flexible and relevant during any stage of drug treatment (e.g., treatment initiation, maintenance, and relapse prevention). For example, in the context of pharmacotherapy, behavioral treatments have been utilized to increase medication adherence, session attendance, and compliance with other treatment procedures. Note that while progress continues in the development of pharmacotherapies for stimulant dependence, no pharmacological agents are currently approved by the U.S. Food and Drug Administration for the treatment of certain stimulants, such as cocaine or methamphetamine (METH). Therefore, knowing how to effectively implement behavioral treatments is important, as they can serve as primary interventions for stimulant dependence. In this chapter, we provide a background and introduction to four common and effective behavioral-based interventions for stimulant dependence: contingency management (CM), cognitive-behavioral therapy (CBT), and group counseling.

Contingency Management

CM treatments are firmly based on extensive behavioral studies illustrating the power of reinforcers to shape and maintain behavior. Reinforcers consist of environmental events (presentation of a stimulus, access to specific activities) that increase the frequency or probability of a response occurring that produced that environmental event. Most organisms are biologically predisposed to treat certain events as reinforcers, such as food and sex, as well as drugs. For example, numerous laboratory studies have demonstrated that animals will self-administer virtually every drug humans are known to commonly abuse. Importantly, laboratory studies in both animals and humans have demonstrated that responding for drugs can be altered by presenting alternative reinforcers. Therefore, CM procedures seek to alter drug-related behaviors by carefully presenting alternative reinforcers for non-drug-related behaviors.

A substantial problem in the treatment of stimulant dependence is how to compete against the relatively immediate and potent reinforcing effects of drug consumption. Benefits of remaining abstinent (e.g., financial stability, better health) may take months or even years to become salient to a given client. CM interventions can bridge this temporal gap by providing frequent alternative reinforcers for remaining drug abstinent. In doing so, CM procedures effectively bolster clients' motivation (which can vary substantially during a quit attempt) to not use drugs.

The efficacy of CM for treating a wide variety of drug use disorders, including stimulant dependence, has been tested and demonstrated in numerous randomized clinical trials (Lussier et al. 2006). CM interventions are extremely flexible in terms of what behaviors can be addressed and how. However, most CM procedures generally have the following components in common (Table 4–1): 1) identifying a target behavior, 2) verifying the target behavior through an objective assessment, 3) choosing an appropriate reinforcer, and 4) planning an effective method for delivering or withholding reinforcers based on the client's performance.

Identifying the Target Behavior

The most common target behavior in CM treatments for drug use is abstinence. However, abstinence can be defined in various ways, and treatment providers must carefully consider these prior to implementing CM. For example, abstinence may be defined episodically, as in the case of a single clinic visit. Alternatively, definitions of abstinence that cover longer durations, such as 1 week or across three consecutive clinic visits, may be used. As longer durations of continuous abstinence during CM treatment are a potent

TABLE 4–1. Overview of contingency management

Identifying target behavior	Drug abstinence
	Session attendance
	Medication compliance
Assessing target behavior	Self-report
	Visual confirmation
	Immunoassay test strips
Choosing an appropriate reinforcer	Money
	Vouchers
	Access to privileges
Delivering reinforcers	Escalating schedule
	Resets
	Prize bowl

predictor of posttreatment abstinence (Higgins et al. 2000), one may be tempted to focus on definitions of abstinence spanning longer durations of time. However, while longer durations of drug abstinence are an important treatment goal, one potential pitfall of choosing to exclusively reinforce a relatively demanding target behavior is that clients may be unable to reach these goals and not earn incentives, especially early during treatment. Subsequently, they may become frustrated and even drop out of treatment. As a hypothetical example, imagine the target behavior is to display abstinence every day for a week, with reinforcement being delivered on the final day. If the participant uses drugs early in the week, let us suppose even the first day, treatment providers lose the ability to provide motivation to remain abstinent for the rest of the week.

The following potential solutions are designed to merely illustrate the flexibility CM provides in tackling such problems. Regardless of the solution chosen, the criterion for obtaining reinforcement should be clearly outlined to clients prior to initiating treatment. As one possible solution, treatment providers can reinforce both single occurrences of abstinence and longer durations of abstinence. This method may minimize potential frustration by providing reinforcement for a relatively simple target behavior while concurrently providing clients the opportunity to receive reinforcement for meeting more demanding target behaviors (Figure 4–1, *left*). A second possible solution is to change the definition of the target behavior over the course of treatment. For example, the target behavior may initially be defined as 1 day of drug abstinence at the beginning of a treatment regimen and increased to 1 week of abstinence as the goals of treatment change over time (Figure 4–1, *right*).

CM procedures can also promote other treatment goals in lieu of or in conjunction with abstinence. In certain situations, treatment providers may wish to reinforce session attendance in order to administer various treatment services regardless of drug-use status. Additionally, stimulant-dependent clients often have additional obstacles in their lives that can interfere with treatment, particularly among those with cocaine or METH dependence. Under such circumstances, treatment providers may choose to reinforce adaptive target behaviors, such as writing a job application, scheduling an appointment with a social worker, meeting court appointments, or engaging in non-drug-related social activities.

Another common target behavior is medication compliance, as compliance is generally poor among those with stimulant dependence. Possible medications of interest include those targeting drug use as well as other conditions commonly associated with drug-using populations (HIV, psychiatric disorders). In regard to medications targeting drug use, CM is particularly helpful in cases where the individual is reluctant to start a first-line medication treatment because the medication may decrease the reinforcing effects of drug consumption or even produce aversive consequences. For example, for some individuals, cocaine use occurs primarily following alcohol consumption. An effective pharmacological treatment for such clients is to administer disulfiram (Antabuse), which interferes with alcohol metabolism. Drinking alcohol after disulfiram administration produces highly unpleasant physiological effects such as dizziness and nausea. Predictably, clients may avoid disulfiram treatment in order to avoid such effects, despite the overall benefits they would gain from not drinking alcohol and subsequently avoiding cocaine.

Some clients may also have difficulty maintaining medication regimens even if the medication does not alter the effects of their drug of choice. For example, the prevalence of HIV is significantly greater among individuals with stimulant dependence relative to the general population, and the HIV infection can develop into AIDS without appropriate treatment. Fortunately, medications mitigating the progression of HIV into AIDS are available, but their success relies on adherence to HIV medication regimens. Similarly, stimulant-dependent individuals have relatively higher occurrences of various psychiatric illnesses for which symptoms can be greatly ameliorated by prescribed medications if they are taken regularly. Despite the benefits of taking HIV and psychiatric medications, individuals may find side effects unpleasant or even simply forget to take their medication. For both these examples, CM procedures can increase the likelihood that individuals maintain their medication regimens.

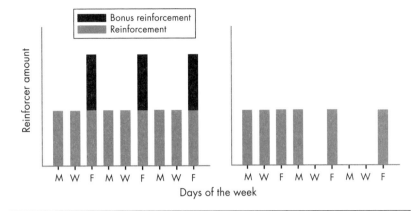

FIGURE 4–1. Example of reinforcing different target behaviors over 3 weeks. Left panel illustrates reinforcers delivered for single occurrences of abstinence (*gray bars*) and bonus for 1 week of abstinence (*black above gray*). Right panel illustrates less frequent reinforcers delivered after longer durations of abstinence.

While the foregoing examples illustrate CM's flexibility in regard to the range of addressable target behaviors, it is important to note the specificity of CM as well. For instance, improved session attendance or medication compliance is associated with increased abstinence. However, if the primary goal is to increase abstinence, reinforcement should be provided directly for abstinence, rather than rewards given for attendance or medication compliance in the hope of obtaining indirect downstream effects on drug use.

Verifying the Target Behavior

After identifying the target behavior, treatment providers must consider how to measure its occurrence. Certain behaviors such as session attendance are relatively easy to assess. Abstinence, on the other hand, requires additional considerations by treatment providers. On one end of the continuum, treatment providers could simply ask clients about their recent drug use. However, even without explicit consequences for drug use, clients often underreport their drug use when verified against biochemical assessments. Under the context of CM, clients have even greater reason to falsely report abstinence, because of incentives. Unfortunately, self-report in this context can potentially have the unintended consequence of reinforcing drug use. Therefore, despite its simplicity, self-report is not an optimal measure of abstinence in the context of CM.

On the other end of the continuum, the gold standard for drug testing includes sophisticated laboratory equipment (i.e., gas chromatography, mass spectrometry) capable of identifying the presence and quantity of specific drug compounds. While such methods are attractive, they are not without their own potential limitations, with the foremost being high cost, which is likely prohibitive for most groups outside of well-funded research studies and hospitals. Costs can be decreased by sending samples out to be analyzed by private groups, but obtaining results from such tests can take weeks. Such delays are undesirable in the context of CM, where immediate feedback is a critical determinant of treatment success. Indeed, a meta-analysis identified immediacy of reinforcement as one of two significant moderators of CM efficacy (Lussier et al. 2006).

Immunoassay tests are an attractive compromise between the two extremes described above. Immunoassays are biochemical tests measuring the presence or concentration of drug metabolites in urine, saliva, or blood and are often used in drug research studies as well as treatment settings. A variety of affordable immunoassay tests exist to fit the specific needs of a given treatment. Different types of immunoassay tests provide qualitative (abstinent or not abstinent), quantitative, or semiquantitative information. Immunoassay tests also range in what kind of drugs they test for (single drug or multiple drugs), and they provide relatively fast results (usually within a few minutes), allowing the care provider to give the client immediate feedback. Finally, immunoassay tests are portable, allowing care providers to conduct tests in nonclinic locations such as the client's home.

Once a specific test for abstinence is selected, care providers need to be aware of how often assessments of abstinence will need to be conducted, particularly if they are interested in accurately assessing continuous abstinence. The frequency of assessment required can be determined by confirming the half-life of a drug or its metabolites. While the half-life of a drug will aid care providers in determining the minimal frequency of assessments, it does not necessarily dictate how often clinic sessions have to be scheduled. In some cases, care providers may wish to schedule more frequent visits to provide additional support and the opportunity to earn incentives as needed by their population of interest.

While frequent clinic visits allow for regular monitoring of drug use as well as opportunities to reinforce abstinence, too frequent visits may be prohibitive. Clients may find it difficult to visit the clinic on a regular basis, and more frequent visits add extra demands on treatment providers and staff. Web-based CM procedures offer a promising innovative answer to such problems. Web-based CM-based treatments were pioneered for the treatment of cigarette smoking (Dallery and Glenn 2005). Smokers were provided with portable breath carbon monoxide (CO) monitors that are used to assess recent smoking. A combination of CO monitors, webcams, and secure Web-based servers was used several times a day to assess clients' smoking status. Of course, additional issues are present when conducting urine-based assessments. However, Web-based CM would be ideal in the case of medication compliance and allows treatment providers to reach clients who do not have ready means of transportation or those who live far away from the clinic.

Choosing Reinforcers

Reinforcers are the driving force behind CM's efficacy in promoting healthy behavior changes. Therefore, care providers need to take special care in choosing an effective as well as appropriate incentive. Specific incentives may function as effective reinforcers for some clients but not necessarily others. Even incentives that are effective at one point in time for a given individual may not be later on. For example, food is an effective reinforcer in hungry organisms, but food's reinforcing value decreases dramatically when animals are full. Ideally, care providers should use flexible reinforcers that are not tied to a specific individual need and are therefore more likely to remain effective across changing conditions. For most people, money is an ideal reinforcer, as it can readily procure a wide variety of goods and services. However, money may pose special concerns in stimulant-dependent populations, where possession of disposable cash may potentially lead to purchasing of drugs and relapse.

An innovative alternative to money is vouchers (Higgins et al. 1993). Voucher-based incentives represent a flexible treatment-based currency system exchangeable for a wide variety of goods and services and are the most commonly used reinforcers in CM-based treatments for stimulant dependence. Vouchers can be delivered in a variety of forms, including gift cards or checks to pay for bills. Implementation of vouchers in CM treatments has several attractive features. For one, they are tied to a range of reinforcers and therefore more likely to retain their reinforcing value regardless of changing conditions. However, treatment providers can exercise a certain degree of control as to the types of goods and services for which vouchers can be exchanged, and thereby can reduce the likelihood that vouchers will be used to obtain inappropriate goods and services such as drugs. Also, voucher-based incentives provide care providers an opportunity to interact with clients to choose appropriate yet still rewarding goals in conjunction with CM treatment. For example, a client may wish to increase healthy behaviors and join a gym. The client's interest in gym membership would represent an opportunity in which the treatment provider could go over the cost of the membership and how to cover the cost using incentives earned from remaining drug abstinent.

Whereas flexible reinforcers such as money and vouchers are ideal, other reinforcers may also be effective under appropriate circumstances. For example, in residential treatment settings, possible reinforcers include access to privileges such as recreation activities, television, and so forth. Additionally, treatment providers have provided their own "shop," in which various items ranging in value can be bought using tokens earned through CM treatment.

Delivering Reinforcers

Over numerous studies, various procedural manipulations have been identified that increase the effectiveness of CM interventions. Two significant moderators of CM efficacy are reinforcer magnitude and time to reinforcer delivery (Lussier et al. 2006). In other words, reinforcers that are of higher value and delivered more quickly upon occurrence of the target behavior are more effective.

In addition to the magnitude and time to delivery, other important procedural manipulations have been discovered that enhance the efficacy of CM. For example, in an escalating schedule, reinforcement magnitude increases as clients continue to meet the target behavior (Roll et al. 1996). In the case of abstinence, fixed reinforcer values may be easier to implement, but an escalating schedule of reinforcement produces greater durations of continuous abstinence, which is associated with improved posttreatment outcomes (Higgins et al. 2000). In a sense, an escalating schedule increases clients' investment in their own abstinence, as they have more to lose by relapsing the longer they remain abstinent. Along the same vein, CM procedures utilizing an escalating schedule often include a reset component, which resets that value of reinforcement should the client not meet the target behavior. For example, imagine a CM procedure in which the reinforcer value starts at $1 and increases by $1 for each subsequent demonstration of abstinence (Figure 4–2). At $10, the client relapses and therefore does not earn the incentive. Additionally, the next time he or she is abstinent, the incentive value is reset to $1. In order to prevent clients from becoming overly discouraged following a reset, it is not uncommon to return the reinforcer value to that prior to relapse following a set number of instances in which the client meets the abstinence criterion.

Potential Limitations of Contingency Management

The most commonly cited potential limitation of CM treatment is cost. In response, CM-based treatment studies continue to examine optimal methods for delivering available reinforcers to be maximally effective in promoting healthy behaviors. The escalating schedule and reset contingency are helpful by-products of this line of research. However, if overall cost remains a hurdle, a variety of innovative solutions have been developed to decrease the financial burden of CM treatment.

One method for addressing costs while still producing treatment effects is to provide reinforcers intermittently. Such procedures are commonly referred to as "prize bowl"– or "fishbowl"–based CM (Petry and Martin 2002). Clients who

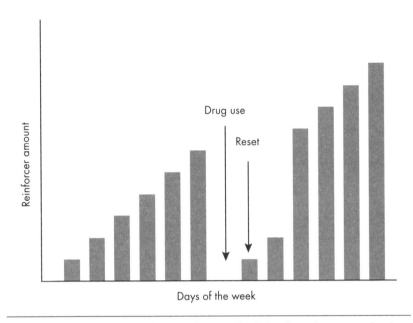

FIGURE 4–2. Example of an escalating schedule of reinforcement for drug abstinence, including a reset in reinforcement amount following drug use.

engage in the target behavior earn the opportunity to draw from a prize bowl. Each draw has the potential to earn prizes of different value, with more expensive prizes being less probable. Most of the draws, however, do not result in an explicit reward. As in more traditional CM interventions, an escalating schedule with resets can also be incorporated, such that continuously meeting the target behavior results in more draws from the prize bowl.

Alternatively, some treatment providers have addressed the cost of CM by seeking help and support directly from the community and local businesses (Garcia-Rodriguez et al. 2008). While this requires additional effort on the part of the treatment provider to contact various agencies, the potential benefit is that all reinforcers may be provided and therefore cost nothing to treatment providers.

Cognitive-Behavioral Therapy

CBT is one of the most widely used and effective forms of psychotherapy for treating stimulant dependence (Lee and Rawson 2008; McHugh et al. 2010). CBT focuses on identification and modification of thoughts and behaviors perpetuating drug use and relapse (Table 4–2). The cognitive aspect of CBT targets individuals' attitudes and beliefs about drug use and abstinence. Treatment is directed at identifying and examining self-defeating or maladaptive thoughts and substituting them with more constructive and healthy ways of viewing oneself and life (Table 4–3). The behavioral aspect of CBT addresses response patterns supporting drug use by replacing them with safer and ultimately more rewarding actions. Such changes are brought about through specific exercises conducted during and between therapy sessions. CBT's focus on a defined problem, structured and short-term approach, and subsequent affordability have made the method popular in research circles, resulting in clearly quantifiable findings, and thus CBT has a broad base of empirical research to support its efficacy.

Strengths of Cognitive-Behavioral Therapy

CBT has a number of benefits that render the modality especially effective for drug-dependent populations. For example, cognitive-behavioral techniques are compatible with many adjunctive treatments. When used in conjunction with medication, CBT has been particularly successful in reducing stimulant use (Carroll et al. 2004; Penberthy et al. 2010). In addition, when used in combination, CBT and CM appear to have a synergistic effect, as CBT has an impact on substance use that tends to increase over time, whereas CM results are more rapidly attained but may be less durable (Rawson 2004). Moreover, CBT can be delivered in an individual or group format (Carroll 1998; Marlatt and Gordon 1985) and in various residential and community-based settings. While the nature of individual therapy lends itself to a more flexible and tailored approach to treatment, a group format provides social support, modeling, and universality. Cognitive-behavioral principles form the basis for the relapse prevention approach (Marlatt and Gordon 1985) and are an integral component of the extensively studied multimodal Matrix model for stimulant abuse (Center for Substance Abuse Treatment 2006). Finally, CBT's methodical approach, while targeting current and pressing problems related to stimulant use, also teaches clients important skills utilizable in other areas of their current and future lives.

Principles of Cognitive-Behavioral Therapy

Social learning theory forms the basis for CBT. The three components utilized are modeling, classical conditioning, and operant conditioning. *Modeling* refers to methods by which individuals learn behaviors by observing

---

TABLE 4–2. Characteristics of cognitive-behavioral therapy for stimulant abuse

---

Based on premise that thoughts are main determinant of feelings and
  actions

Relatively brief (usually 12–16 sessions) and time-limited

Based on collaborative relationship between therapist and client

Structured and goal-oriented

Includes functional analyses of stimulant use

Provides skills training

Has an educational focus (as opposed to "just talking")

Coping skills rehearsed during sessions

Homework assignments given at each session

---

others and subsequently experimenting with the behavior themselves. Just as children become adept at tying their shoes by watching their parents, stimulant users may commence drug use after observing their friends use drugs. In the context of CBT sessions, the therapist models, through role-play, effective ways of managing cravings, solving problems, using refusal skills, and dealing with other issues related to drug use. The client in turn rehearses these skills during sessions and implements them in day-to-day life.

Classical conditioning describes the process by which a formerly neutral stimulus can provoke a conditioned response after repeated pairing with an unconditioned stimulus. In the case of drugs, stimulant use may be associated with particular cues (i.e., people, places, and things) over time, so that eventually many components of one's environment evoke powerful urges that frequently lead to drug use. Through explanation of this concept over the course of CBT, the nature of the client's strong cravings may to some extent become demystified. Clients are also taught that conditioned responses (cravings for drug) will extinguish through recurrent exposure to conditioned stimuli (environmental cues) in the absence of unconditioned stimuli (effects of drug consumption).

According to the principles of operant conditioning, reinforced behaviors occur with greater frequency. It follows that stimulant use and correlated behaviors are learned through pairing with pleasurable qualities of the drugs and association with external stimuli. The purpose of CBT is to weaken these learned associations by analyzing consequences maintaining drug use, modifying behavior accordingly, and substituting drug use with appropriate non-drug-related activities.

Roles of Therapist and Client in Cognitive-Behavioral Therapy

The CBT therapist serves as a coach, educator, and model. During the initial session, the therapist focuses on developing a rapport with the client, teaching the principles of CBT, learning the client's current and specific reasons for seeking treatment, and inquiring as to the client's strengths and sources of support. The therapist is then in a position to tailor his or her instruction, modeling, and encouragement of the client in effective ways of achieving and maintaining abstinence. As treatment progresses, the therapist continues to strive for a balance between presenting the pertinent didactic material, assigning homework, and maintaining an effective collaborative bond with the client. The therapist praises attempts by the client to apply coping skills and offers a nonjudgmental, problem-solving response with constructive criticism when such attempts fall short of the client's aim.

The client learns how to perform functional analyses and various new coping skills with the therapist during each treatment session. In addition, the client practices these strategies in his or her day-to-day life, completes homework exercises, and reports back to the therapist regarding implementation of the newly acquired skills, along with drug-use status. Many drug users feel empowered and relieved by CBT's premise that people can change if they choose to and put forth the effort. The therapist points out that over time the individual has practiced and thus learned certain ways of reacting to situations, both cognitively and behaviorally. The client has thus demonstrated that he or she is capable of learning specific skills, in this case related to stimulant use, and in a similar way can unlearn detrimental "skills" and learn more adaptive behaviors. However, in order for treatment to be effective and the results to be long-lasting, the client must also embrace the principle of practice and repetition of the new cognitive and behavioral techniques. The weekly homework assignments underscore the clearly structured goals of CBT for the stimulant-dependent individual.

Main Components of Cognitive-Behavioral Therapy

The main components of CBT consist of a *functional analysis* and *skills training*. Overall, a functional analysis identifies variables maintaining drug use by examining situations in which such use is likely to occur, thoughts and feelings that occurred during the drug-use episode, the behaviors the client engaged in, and the consequences of his or her behavior. During the first therapy session, an in-depth functional analysis is conducted investigating the client's history and

TABLE 4–3. Revising cognitive distortions

Maladaptive/ self-defeating thought	Constructive thought/ behavior
I have to… I should… I must… I ought to…	I choose to… It would be advisable, preferable, helpful, to my advantage…
I can't stand this [anxiety, depression, loneliness, boredom, anger] one more minute.	I'm uncomfortable right now, but this won't last forever. I can handle this. I accept that I'm uncomfortable at this moment. This too shall pass. How can I make the best of the situation? —I can call a friend. —I can look at my list of pleasurable activities and pick one to do. —I can take some slow, deep breaths, count to ten, and calm myself.
My life is a nightmare.	I'm going through a difficult time, but I have coping skills with which to deal with this.
It's wrong for me to feel [anxious, depressed, lonely, bored, angry]. I should always be happy and positive.	Everyone experiences painful feelings at times. I'm only human, just like everyone else.
I've never been able to quit drug use before. Trying to quit is impossible.	With practice and perseverance, change is possible. The only way to fail is to no longer try.
I slipped and used today. This proves that I'm hopeless.	I can learn from this experience and make changes so that this doesn't have to happen again.
I'm feeling worse now that I'm abstinent than when I was using.	Letting go of a substance is causing my body to go through a lot of changes. This won't last forever.
Practicing new thoughts and behaviors is difficult.	Yes, trying new things feels awkward at first, but in time this will seem more natural, and my current methods aren't working for me.
I don't want to…	I don't need to wait until I want to do something in order to do it. Often, changing my behavior can lead to my feeling differently.

current pattern of stimulant use and how these have affected various areas of his or her life (e.g., relationships, vocation, finances). The client is then expected to conduct several written functional analyses between sessions, for episodes of drug craving during that week, and to bring these assessments to subsequent therapy sessions to be reviewed with the therapist. Functional analyses, also known as the "thoughts, feelings, and behaviors" worksheet (Figure 4–3), are thus a continual part of the treatment process.

During skills training, clients are taught healthy and adaptive coping skills not involving drug use. By the time individuals reach the point of seeking treatment for drug dependence, they often have come to rely on drugs as their primary method for dealing with problems. As a result, the client's ability to utilize non-drug-related coping skills may have atrophied or never adequately developed. In CBT, clients are expected to learn, practice, and consequently strengthen a wide variety of coping strategies. In terms of drug use, CBT offers three strategies: *recognize* a potentially dangerous situation, *avoid* such situations whenever possible, and *cope* when avoidance is impossible or inappropriate.

Setting for Cognitive-Behavioral Therapy

As a general rule, CBT is conducted on an outpatient basis, as this allows the client and therapist the best opportunity to evaluate what factors in the client's everyday life continue to contribute to stimulant use. In addition, as an outpatient the client is afforded the opportunity to practice the skills learned during sessions in real-life circumstances. At the next therapy session, the client and therapist can then discuss what techniques were and were not effective and how to modify the client's coping strategies during similar situations in the future.

Primary Aims of Cognitive-Behavioral Therapy

Over the course of CBT for stimulant use, the following issues are addressed: 1) clarifying triggers for drug use through functional analyses; 2) managing cravings; 3) cultivating effective drug-refusal techniques; 4) developing problem-solving skills; 5) developing coping skills for emergencies; 6) improving decision-making skills; and 7) tolerating uncomfortable feelings, thoughts, and bodily sensations.

As described earlier (see subsection "Main Components of Cognitive-Behavioral Therapy"), functional analyses are conducted at the initial session, during subsequent sessions, and between sessions, to determine the prime factors driving the client's craving for stimulants. An examination of the pros and cons of continued drug use is conducted. The participant is re-

Functional Analysis				
Trigger	**Thoughts and feelings**	**Behavior**	**Positive consequences**	**Negative consequences**
What set me up to use?	What was I thinking? What was I feeling?	What did I do then?	What positive things happened?	What negative things happened?
A friend offered me some meth at a party.	A little bit won't hurt me. I'm feeling kind of down, and this will help me enjoy myself.	Used meth.	I felt more energetic, talkative, and happier for a while.	When I came down, I felt more depressed than ever. I'd also promised my partner that I wouldn't use again, and now I either have to lie to him or tell him the truth, and he'll be disappointed in me.

FIGURE 4–3. Example of a functional analysis, also known as the "thoughts, feelings, and behaviors" worksheet.

spected as an individual who makes the decisions and takes responsibility for his or her life. It is often helpful for the client to list on the front of an index card the perceived pros of quitting drug use, and on the back the cons of continuing to use; the client can keep this card in his or her wallet for reference during a difficult moment of drug craving (Figure 4–4).

While the therapist makes it clear that abstinence remains the goal of treatment, the therapist also conveys that not all people achieve abstinence instantaneously and that it is an ongoing process. This explanation can circumvent the "abstinence violation effect," in which an individual becomes discouraged by an episode of drug use or "slip" while in treatment and proceeds into full relapse. In CBT, slips, while not ideal, are seen as valuable opportunities to learn. Just as a child learns to walk by first crawling, then standing, taking tentative steps, inevitably falling, standing up, and trying again, the client who is undergoing treatment for stimulant use should be encouraged to persevere and recognize that slips are sometimes part of the recovery process and can be viewed as a learning experience (i.e., as "information, not ammunition").

Craving for one's stimulant of choice during initial and prolonged abstinence can feel overwhelming and perhaps insurmountable for many stimulant-dependent individuals. The therapist can offer reassurance by explaining that the phenomenon of craving is normal and that it is not a reflection on the client's ability or desire to quit drug use. Using learning theory, the therapist explains that over time, as the participant has turned to drug use in a variety of situations, many activities have become associated with drug use, and thus craving is to be expected. However, it is also emphasized that craving is time-limited, provided that the client does not engage in drug use. So the answer is not to eliminate the craving but to learn methods by which to manage the craving without resorting to drug use.

Such methods can include distracting oneself, talking about the craving with a trusted individual, experiencing the craving without struggling or acquiescing to it, remembering the deleterious results of drug use, using encouraging and realistic self-talk, and compiling a list of pleasurable or rewarding activities that do not include drug use, to be scheduled regularly into the client's life as well as during moments of drug craving. If the client expresses difficulty tolerating uncomfortable emotions, such feelings can be normalized. Accepting difficult feelings can be compared to the building of a muscle, which may become sore after a strenuous workout but will ultimately become stronger as a result of continued exercise. The in-session practice techniques and homework assignments can feel awkward at times, but perseverance will eventually lead to enhanced coping skills for the client. The therapist can emphasize that the only failure is to no longer try.

In addition, the therapist coaches the client in decreasing contact with high-risk individuals, objects, or situations. Examples include getting rid of paraphernalia (e.g., lighters, syringes) and reducing or preferably eliminating contact with drug-using friends, which may involve deleting phone numbers of such individuals from one's cell phone or changing one's phone number. Other strategies are meeting friends at a coffee shop rather than a bar and altering routines. For instance, if a client associates using stimulants with the end of the workday and spending time with certain acquaintances on Fridays, he or she can be coached in developing an alternative activity for Friday evenings in the near future. Clients are also taught that HALT (being Hungry, Angry, Lonely, or Tired) can serve as a trigger and to utilize coping strategies to avoid or ameliorate these feeling states.

Since the client may still have contact with people who may offer him or her drugs, the therapist gives suggestions as to how the client can cultivate effective drug-refusal skills. Options include giving a prompt and clear response that the client is no longer using drugs, making a respectful request that the other person not offer the client drugs on future occasions, and changing the subject of conversation. The client and therapist then practice role-plays in anticipation of such a situation, during which the client can be coached in the difference between passive, assertive, and aggressive responses.

Pros of stimulant abstinence
I'll feel better about myself.
My partner will be happy.
I'll save money.
My health will be better.
I'll avoid possible run-ins with the law.
I'll learn to tolerate my feelings and face my problems directly.

Cons of using stimulants
I'll feel disappointed in myself.
My partner will be angry.
Cost.
My health will suffer.
I could be arrested.
I might get caught up in a pattern of using regularly again.
When I come down, I'll feel even worse.

FIGURE 4–4. Example of an index card listing the perceived pros of quitting drug use on one side and cons of continuing to use on the other, which the client can keep in his or her wallet for reference during a difficult moment of drug craving.

While cessation of drug use is the immediate goal of therapy and will ultimately aid in the client's ability to cope with life, in the short run drug abstinence usually forces the client to directly face many issues he or she had swept under the rug while using. The client's resultant anxiety or depression can be made all the more acute by the client's not using drugs to ameliorate his or her disquieting feelings. In addition, the cognitive difficulties often experienced in early abstinence from stimulant use can compound the client's ability to come up with effective solutions to various problems. Thus, the outlining and rehearsal of a structured, straightforward approach to solving problems can be very helpful, in which the therapist guides the client to acknowledge the problem, identify and clarify the problem, and brainstorm potential solutions. The client then selects the approach deemed most likely to succeed, attempts the selected approach and judges its effectiveness, and modifies the plan as needed.

To develop coping skills for emergencies, the therapist asks the client to list several significantly stressful events that may occur in the near future and how these might impact the client's grip on abstinence. The therapist and client then formulate clear action plans to cope with these potential stressors. Lists can be developed, with phone numbers of supportive people, distracting and safe activities, and constructive thoughts to counter dangerous thoughts about drug use. The client can also keep handwritten reminders regarding the destructive consequences of relapsing into drug use and safe locations to endure the difficult episode.

Stimulant-dependent individuals may often minimize the impact that their seemingly inconsequential, everyday decisions can have on their ability to achieve and maintain abstinence from drug use. However, a choice that on the surface seems unrelated to drug use can make the difference between a slip into drug use and the maintenance of abstinence. For example, the client may relate that over the weekend he was missing a friend with whom he used to take drugs on occasion, so the client decided to call the friend "just to say hi." This led to the friend inviting the client over, offering the client drugs, and the client succumbing to temptation. The therapist points out how the seemingly irrelevant decision to contact the friend jeopardized the client's abstinence, and coaches the client in improving his decision-making skills. Examples of less risky decisions include calling a friend who does not use drugs, distracting oneself by getting busy with an endeavor on one's list of rewarding activities, or simply tolerating the loneliness for a while and knowing that "this too shall pass."

CBT for stimulant use also often includes mindfulness training. Defined as nonjudgmental awareness of the present moment, mindfulness techniques teach clients to change their attitude or relationship toward uncomfortable feelings, thoughts, or physical sensations through observing such experiences without reacting. For example, clients can be instructed to picture their mind as a blue sky. One's thoughts can be likened to clouds that move through the sky and are thus temporary. Another example is "urge surfing." When experiencing a craving to use drugs, the client learns to imagine the urge as a wave, which eventually crests, breaks, and then disperses. In a similar manner, clients can "go with the flow" of an urge, learning that the urge will dissipate over time and that the client can survive without acting out on the impulse to use stimulants. Simultaneously, clients are encouraged to modify their actions as appropriate. Thus, acceptance of one's situation does not imply a passive stance in regard to one's life. Instead, as a result of increased awareness and tolerance of the present moment, clients become more adept at making constructive behavioral changes rather than acting on "automatic pilot."

Structure of Therapy Sessions

The usual length of CBT treatment for stimulant use ranges from 12 to 16 weeks and includes an average of 12 sessions, which are typically 60 minutes in length for individual sessions and 90 minutes for a group format. The amount of didactic material to be presented during sessions necessitates that the therapist stay on task while also maintaining receptivity and flexibility should the client require more or less time on a particular topic. Accordingly, for individual treatment, CBT sessions are generally divided into a 20/20/20 sequence for the therapeutic hour.

During the first 20 minutes, the client discusses his or her experience with the homework assignment from the previous session, any episodes of drug craving or use, and coping strategies employed since the past session. The therapist praises the client's completion of homework assignments, if applicable. In the event that the client did not attempt the homework or found it difficult to do, the therapist and client generate ways that the client can deal with such obstacles in the future, and the therapist points out that individuals who spend time on the homework have greater chances of recovery.

During the next 20 minutes, the therapist introduces the next topic and assigns a new homework exercise. It is important that the therapist provide a clear rationale for the new skill. For instance, the therapist may say,

> You mentioned that since stopping cocaine use you've felt bored, since you're not spending a lot of time trying to get cocaine, using it, and recovering from the results. The good news is that you have a lot more time on your hands. However, it's important to fill some of that time with constructive activities that are also pleasurable for you, so you aren't tempted to break your abstinence. Let's start a list of some safe and enjoyable events you can do if you're bored. On your own, you can continue adding to this list over the next week and try one or more of these activities if boredom strikes.

Thus, the therapist relates the current assignment to the client's current concerns and enhances the client's motivation to complete the exercise.

The final 20 minutes of the session are devoted to discussing how the client can utilize the new exercise or other coping skills in anticipated high-risk situations over the next week. The client can relate any concerns or confusion regarding the assignment, which the therapist then attempts to alleviate. The therapist also reiterates his or her belief in the client's ability to successfully meet upcoming challenges, while also tempering overconfidence that might cause the client to unnecessarily expose himself or herself to perilous circumstances.

Limitations of Cognitive-Behavioral Therapy

For all of CBT's attributes, the method does have some limitations. First of all, the many strategies employed in CBT make it somewhat cumbersome to train clinicians in administering the treatment effectively. In general, a 2-day to 1-week didactic seminar is recommended, along with case supervision, a master's degree in psychology or an associated mental health field, 3 years of experience with a substance abuse population, and some familiarity with

CBT principles and techniques. The likelihood is high that in many communities, the number of such adequately trained professionals will not be sufficient to treat all clients who seek face-to-face therapy.

Furthermore, CBT requires an adequate level of cognitive ability on the part of the client, at the very time when the client may be struggling with cognitive difficulties in the early stages of abstinence from a stimulant. Cognitive hurdles may be ameliorated through the use of medications in conjunction with CBT. In addition, the therapist's paying close attention to the client's understanding of material presented during sessions and ability to carry out homework assignments can minimize the impact of cognitive challenges on the effectiveness of CBT. However, the pacing of face-to-face sessions may still present difficulties.

In addition, CBT, as well as other face-to-face psychotherapeutic modalities, can be time-consuming for both the client and therapist. Scheduling appointments can also pose problems, along with transportation to the therapy site. Additionally, some clients remain wary of the stigma associated with seeing a therapist.

Computerized Cognitive-Behavioral Therapy

Internet-delivered CBT has been investigated as a solution to these challenges of face-to-face therapy sessions, with favorable results for a variety of health conditions (Cuijpers et al. 2008), including substance abuse (Amstadter et al. 2009). Given the inherently structured format of CBT, the development of computer-based programs with clearly defined therapeutic modules and assignments does not pose a challenge. In the present computer age, the majority of people are familiar and comfortable with the basic operations of a computer, and Web-based programs can be tailored to include graphics and animations that enhance the appeal of the sessions and homework. Furthermore, computer-administered modules can offer immediate and objective feedback to clients regarding their level of understanding and ability to implement the treatment strategies presented, so that clients may be able to pace themselves accordingly and review the session material if needed. In areas where mental health professionals with suitable qualifications are not available, Web-based CBT can fill this practitioner gap, in addition to computer-based CBT being attractive from a financial standpoint (Carroll et al. 2008).

The effects of Internet-administered CBT appear to last over time. In a study by Carroll et al. (2008), substance users who were assigned to six modules of computer-assisted delivery of CBT (CBT4CBT) had significantly larger reductions in number of drug-positive urine samples and had generally longer periods of abstinence than clients assigned to treatment as usual.

Moreover, by 6-month follow-up, most individuals assigned to CBT4CBT had continued to improve (Carroll et al. 2009). Hence, computerized CBT appears to result in both short-term and sustained reduction of substance use. However, it is important to note that in this study, all participants, including those assigned to CBT4CBT, received substantial drug counseling, as well as urine testing twice a week during the active portion of the study, suggesting that computerized CBT may be best implemented in a multimodal treatment plan, rather than as a stand-alone approach.

Further studies have lent credence to a therapist-assisted Internet-delivered form of CBT (Kay-Lambkin 2008; Vernmark et al. 2010), demonstrating that face-to-face therapy sessions remain a valuable and frequently indispensable component of treatment for a number of clients. Some individuals may value the in-person connection with a therapist, for motivational and interpersonal purposes. Considering that much communication is nonverbal, a face-to-face session with a therapist also allows the therapist the opportunity to pick up on nonverbal cues, such as vocal inflection and appearance of the client. Likewise, the physical presence and nonverbal cues of the therapist can serve as a model to the client. Thus, a hybrid of computer-based and in-person therapist-assisted treatment may be the most efficacious method in which to deliver therapy for some clients, and it may behoove the therapist or mental health clinic to maintain this treatment option.

Group Counseling

Among the behavioral treatments discussed in the current chapter, group-based therapies have the longest tradition and are arguably still the most common treatment for those with drug dependence. Compared with individual treatment approaches, group counseling programs offer individuals social support and empathy from those with similar experiences. A range of programs are available for individuals with stimulant dependence that provide a variety of services and support not only for clients but their friends and family members as well. The most prominent forms of group therapy are 12-step programs, CBT group approaches, and psychodynamic group approaches. While many group therapies share features of each approach, it is helpful to go over the defining characteristics of each treatment.

12-Step Programs

The original 12-step program, Alcoholics Anonymous, was founded in 1935 by Bill Wilson and Dr. Bob Smith. Since then, 12-step programs have flourished. Alcoholics Anonymous remains the largest of the 12-step programs, followed by Narcotics Anonymous, which was formed to address drug dependence not specifically related to alcohol. Additionally, stimulant-dependent clients may also attend groups held by Cocaine Anonymous and Crystal Meth Anonymous.

The first 12-step programs were based on a model of a Christian fellowship, although more recent forms have made alterations to language specific to religion. Defining characteristics of the actual 12 steps (Table 4–4) consist of the following: admitting that one is powerless against drugs and that control should therefore be passed on to a higher power; careful self-examination and acknowledgment of one's faults and defects, which includes confronting and making amends to those who have been injured in the past; and working with others to move through the 12 steps of the program. Individuals who have completed the 12 steps can act as sponsors to newer members in the program. Members who continue to have problems with drug use are encouraged to increase their involvement in the group or fellowship activities and continue working through the 12 steps.

Relative to the other approaches, 12-step programs are potentially more confrontational, particularly under circumstances in which the individual is in denial in regard to the severity of his or her own drug use. Additionally, an underlying and guiding assumption of 12-step programs is that addiction is a disease that can be controlled but never cured. Therefore, there are no acceptable levels of use for even legal drugs such as alcohol. Since addiction is a chronic disease that the individual cannot control on his or her own, 12-step programs emphasize relinquishing control over to a higher power such as God or the group itself. A general solution to continuing drug-related problems is greater immersion into activities of the 12-step program.

Cognitive-Behavioral Therapy Group Counseling Approaches

CBT group counseling shares many characteristics with CBT for individuals. The defining characteristics of CBT are covered elsewhere in this chapter (see section "Cognitive-Behavioral Therapy"), but it is worth reiterating the primary characteristics of CBT. First, drug use is assumed to be a learned behavior, and clients are taught how to identify antecedents and consequences of their drug use by conducting a functional analysis. Through such exercises, clients are taught how to avoid situations in which they are likely to use drugs, how to cope with cravings, and how to seek healthy alternatives to using drugs. Clients are also provided educational information regarding their drug use. For example, clients may learn about the health conse-

---

TABLE 4–4. The 12 Steps

Step

1. We admitted we were powerless over our addiction—that our lives had become unmanageable.

2. Came to believe a Power greater than ourselves could restore us to sanity.

3. Made a decision to turn our will and our lives over to the care of God as we understood Him.

4. Made a searching and fearless moral inventory of ourselves.

5. Admitted to God, to ourselves, and to another human being the exact nature of our wrongs.

6. Were entirely ready to have God remove all these defects of character.

7. Humbly asked Him to remove our shortcomings.

8. Made a list of all persons we had harmed, and became willing to make amends to them all.

9. Made direct amends to such people wherever possible, except when to do so would injure them or others.

10. Continued to take personal inventory and when we were wrong promptly admitted it.

11. Sought through prayer and meditation to improve our conscious contact with God as we understood Him, praying only for knowledge of His will for us and the power to carry that out.

12. Having had a spiritual awakening as the result of these Steps, we tried to carry this message to alcoholics, and to practice these principles in all our affairs.

Source. Alcoholics Anonymous: *Alcoholics Anonymous: The Story of How Many Thousands of Men and Women Have Recovered From Alcoholism.* New York, Alcoholics Anonymous World Services, Inc., 1993.

quences of continued use as well as the benefits of quitting. Clients may also learn what to expect in terms of withdrawal and craving should they decide to quit.

Similar to 12-step approaches, CBT group counseling follows a structured series of steps, although the actual steps may not be as well defined as those of 12-step programs. In contrast to 12-step programs, CBT group counseling interprets drug use as a learned behavior rather than a chronic, untreatable condition. Therefore, greater emphasis is placed on avoiding drug use triggers, learning why an individual uses drugs, and finding suitable alternatives to replace drug use. In this sense, 12-step programs teach individuals to relinquish control, whereas CBT approaches emphasize techniques to improve self-control. Note that neither approach is necessarily better, and the ultimate utility likely resides in the needs of the individual.

Psychodynamic Group Counseling

The psychodynamic approach to drug use views drug use as a symptom of some unresolved, underlying problem. From this perspective, individuals may be using drugs as a form of self-medication to find relief from suffering and distress related to negative emotional states, feelings of poor self-worth, and destructive relationships with others. Therefore, drug use is treated by first identifying and treating these unresolved issues. The underlying causes of drug use are uncovered through an exploratory process. Critical to the exploratory process is the group, which provides a safe, structured, and supportive environment that allows the individual his or her personal vulnerabilities.

In contrast with 12-step and CBT approaches, psychodynamic group counseling is exploratory in nature and is relatively less structured. Psychodynamic group therapy shares with CBT group counseling the view that drug use can be treated and ultimately cured

Motivational Interviewing for Stimulant Abuse and Dependence

Many summaries and training resources are available in print and online to help providers learn about motivational interviewing (MI). A brief description of these resources and where to obtain them is included in Table 4–5.

In the following overview we discuss the use of MI for METH dependence, with an eye toward the unique challenges of treating this substance use disorder. This overview also is aimed at people who are less familiar with and/or may be skeptical about this approach. Use of MI for METH dependence may require more repetitions, more patience, and attention to specific pitfalls. MI for stimulant dependence will most likely be an integrated feature of a comprehensive, long-term program as opposed to a brief, stand-alone intervention.

When you are about to meet with a person who is dependent on METH, what are your goals for the session? What are your usual expectations going into a first session? What should you, or can you, accomplish? How do you know if progress has been made? How do you manage a patient who may be desperate or hostile or extremely depressed or paranoid or manipulative? What if the person does not want treatment? What if the person is already in treatment or already has been treated for METH dependence—how would this affect your strategy? How can you increase this client's motivation?

TABLE 4–5. Learning and training resources for motivational interviewing

---

Web-based resource	http://www.motivationalinterview.org/
Videos	Motivational Interviewing Training Video: A Tool for Learners. To order: http://www.mitrainingvideo.com
	Motivational Interviewing: Professional Training Series Videos http://www.psychotherapy.net/video/miller-motivational-interviewing
Coding instruments	Moyers TB, Martin T, Manuel JK, et al.: Revised Global Scales: Motivational Interviewing Treatment Integrity 3.0 (MITI 3.0) http://casaa.unm.edu/download/miti3_1.pdf
Books	Miller WR, Rollnick S: *Motivational Interviewing: Preparing People for Change,* 2nd Edition. New York, Guilford, 2002
	Arkowitz H, Westra HA, Miller WR, et al. (eds.): *Motivational Interviewing in the Treatment of Psychological Problems.* New York, Guilford, 2008
Meta-analyses	Lundahl B, Burke B: "The Effectiveness and Applicability of Motivational Interviewing: A Practice-Friendly Review of Four Meta-Analyses." *Journal of Clinical Psychology* 65:1232–1245, 2009
	Lundahl BW, Tollefson D, Gambles C, et al.: "A Meta-Analysis of Motivational Interviewing: Twenty-Five Years of Empirical Studies." *Research on Social Work Practice* 20:137–160, 2010

Motivational interviewing is, simply put, a way to talk with clients about change. More specifically, MI is a "directive, client-centered approach to increasing motivation by helping clients resolve ambivalence" (Miller and Rollnick 2002, p. 25). MI is "directive," in that the provider attempts to keep the conversation on target, not directive in the sense of telling a person what to do. So, instead of simply educating clients and warning them about consequences (which they usually already know and are being told by many other sources), an MI approach aims to do something different. The metaphor most commonly used to convey what an MI session looks like or feels like is a dance. If the lead provides the right support and balance, the partner can respond without being pulled over. There are many ways that providers can provoke resistance or reactance to change. MI training helps providers to lead and maintain the balance by using subtle skills.

Two prima facie features of psychotherapeutic interventions for substance use disorders are that they involve interactions between people (therapist and client) and that the behavior to be changed is often incomprehensibly self-destructive, despite the client knowing that it is. Other approaches to treating drug dependence address behavior change via different mechanisms and theoretical viewpoints. MI addresses the influence of the provider on the quality of the interaction between provider and patient and how that interaction affects client behavior. Successful MI practice entails keeping in mind important theories and research findings on interacting with people engaged in self-destructive behavior. MI skills and principles can be seen as *antidotes to reactance, paradoxes of will and choice,* and the *effects of external consequences* that keep people stuck with low levels of motivation.

Brehm (1966; Brehm and Brehm 1981) proposed the theory of *reactance,* arguing that when people perceive a threat to their freedom of choice and self-determination, they experience a negative emotional reaction that leads to anything from defensiveness and strengthening of their commitment to engaging in that behavior, to opposition and outright obstinacy or defiance. This partly explains why people continue to engage in harmful behaviors despite repeated warnings about detrimental consequences. People value self-determination. People retreat when behavior they see as private is criticized and criminalized. MI has extended these ideas to the field of health behavior or lifestyle change. MI insists that most people experience ambivalence when confronted with making major changes in lifestyle, and that ambivalence is normal, not pathological. Thus, central to the MI approach is using techniques to reduce resistance (or reactance) and help clients work through ambivalence. Ambivalence and reactance can be particularly high among people experiencing uncontrollable use of a drug that has hijacked the dopaminergic reward system in the brain and who are experiencing social shame and punishment for using. In an early study of MI, Miller et al. (1993) found that behavior change was much more likely when therapists behaved in a way that did not elicit resistance or defensiveness among clients compared to when therapists took a more confrontational approach. Indeed, findings from Project MATCH (Project MATCH Research Group 1997) found that MI was more effective than CBT for reducing drinking among clients high in anger.

A second important theoretical viewpoint is *cognitive dissonance theory* (Festinger 1957; Festinger and Carlsmith 1959). This theory can account for self-destructive behavior that persists despite knowledge of its consequences. It also provides strategies for intervening. This view proposes that when people become aware of inconsistencies between their values or their beliefs and their behavior, this awareness generates anxiety and people work to reduce that anxiety. Changing one's beliefs is easier than changing behavior, however. So people typically handle discrepancies between self-harming behavior and their view of themselves by altering either their view of themselves or their view of the behavior instead of changing the behavior. Some refer to this as rationalizing. MI addresses this by skillfully calling attention to discrepancies in an environment that is empathic and nonconfrontational so that clients can deal with the daunting task of changing behavior instead.

Willpower, an extension of motivation, is not something a provider can literally give to a client. It seems clear that many typically used strategies—warning, persuading, frightening, penalizing, charging, convicting, shaming, confronting, and so forth—often fail to motivate enough willpower to make clients stop using. Further, these strategies create a context in which users are motivated to hide and minimize their use. Recent advances in psycholinguistics and related research on human cognition and decision making offer guidance about counselor skills, based on insight into the importance of language and self-talk in motivation. For example, Senay et al. (2010) published startling findings demonstrating that repeating self-interrogating statements of will ("Will I? Will I?") as opposed to declarative statements ("I will. I will.") significantly increased performance of the behavior in question (anagram solving). Questioning oneself, paradoxically, may lead to increased motivation because the types of internal responses generated to the question are more affirmative than responses generated to an externally imposed declaration. Further, Senay et al. stated that "the grammatical structure of self-talk can also be activated implicitly" and "merely seeing another person use interrogative self-talk may be enough to produce the same effect" (Senay et al. 2010, p. 503). Thus, the counselor's careful choice of language subtly but powerfully shapes the form of client self-talk. More generally, Amrhein's (2004; Amrhein et al. 2003, 2004) research shows that increases in self-motivational statements in counseling sessions predict decreased use of drugs for some time to come. Importantly, though, Miller et al. (1993) demonstrated that low levels of client resistance are perhaps most important in predicting decreased alcohol use. In this study, MI-based therapy was more successful than a confrontational counseling style in decreasing alcohol misuse.

Many in the substance abuse treatment field are familiar with the Transtheoretical Model, or theory of the Stages of Change (Prochaska and DiClemente 1984; Prochaska et al. 1992). However, data supporting this view have proven elusive (Bridle et al. 2005), and this suggests that motivation is fluid and dynamic and is not easily placed in particular categories (Litrell and Girvin 2002). Most people accept as obvious the idea that some clients clearly are less motivated to stop using than others. MI is clearly most intended for

TABLE 4–6. Summary of spirit, skills, and principles of motivational interviewing

Spirit	Skills	Principles
Collaboration	Open questions	Express empathy
Evocation	Affirmations	Develop discrepancy
Autonomy	Reflective listening	Roll with resistance
	Summarizing	Support self-efficacy

clients with little or unsolidified motivation. MI skills are also still applicable and very useful during the implementation of other interventions, such as CM, CBT, and pharmacotherapy.

Doing good-quality MI requires training to learn the three fundamental elements of MI spirit, the extensive use of four specific skills, and the four main principles of practice (see Table 4–6). The three elements forming the core of the MI approach or "spirit," toward which all skills are in service, are Collaboration, Evocation, and Autonomy. These elements define the overall therapeutic style of MI. The provider's aim is to evoke the client to talk—not provoke. The client needs to talk, or "do the work," in an MI session. To achieve this, the provider needs to use skills shown to facilitate and avoid behaviors that reduce client-talk. Collaboration may be difficult to achieve when the provider perceives the client to be "in denial" or to be "unwilling to see the consequences of his behavior." However, some shifts in the therapist's perspective and strategy can facilitate the client's motivation to do the very difficult work of changing. Evoking client-talk involves conveying that the provider is willing to listen, using strategies that make clients talk, and providing verbal reinforcement of client-talk. Autonomy is critical to the approach not only in that the provider shows respect and accepts that he or she cannot force the client to change, but further to *facilitate* the client's own sense of autonomy. The counselor's job is not to enforce legal consequences, but rather to facilitate the client's awareness of the sources of his or her motivation, and facilitate the client's desire to achieve valued life goals. Autonomy can be facilitated by direct statements, yet the therapist avoids trying to overtly direct client behavior. The goal is an increase in the client's desire to independently choose a healthy path because the client wants it, not because external sources are insisting or persuading. Autonomy over the drug also is something clients struggle to achieve. MI believes people can regain the ability to choose an independent path and achieve self-direction.

MI providers practice and perfect the extensive use of four behaviors or skills, referred to by the acronym OARS: open-ended questions, affirming,

TABLE 4–7. Potential behavior targets of motivational interviewing

1. Maintain treatment
2. Reinitiate treatment
3. Decrease binge use
4. Maintain abstinence
5. Help engage in aspects of a program already enrolled in
6. Target sobriety sampling
7. Target abstinence for a limited amount of time
8. Discuss a positive urine toxicology result
9. Discuss "relapse thoughts"

reflective listening, and summarizing. Because these skills have been summarized many times in other sources, in the present summary we will emphasize the clinical impact that just these four skills can have and put them in context with CM and CBT, the other behavioral approaches discussed in this chapter. It is recommended that interested readers watch video-based training materials to learn more, and take some time to watch videotaped examples and keep a tally of the O's, A's, R's, and S's. Remember that the skills need to be used extensively and repeatedly.

When you read what the four skills are, you may think, "That's it? Those four simple techniques are going to make someone quit using meth?" When you use MI to converse with a client, as with CM, the target behavior requires careful consideration and must be clearly defined. With METH dependence, it is probably unrealistic to expect that the goal of quitting will be the most productive one to choose. Also as described for CM, a specific step or shorter-term goal likely will be more reasonable; discussing immediate, permanent abstinence from METH is likely to be too overwhelming and complicated. The patient's desire to quit may be very strong, but willpower or commitment to action may be serious barriers. The most important thing to consider is that the choice of target behavior must be the client's. The setting in which you are working with the client as well as the client's stage of readiness may influence the target behavior. Some example MI behavior targets to discuss that may correlate with stage of readiness and setting are listed in Table 4–7.

The four principles of practicing MI are to express empathy, develop discrepancy, avoid arguing, and support self-efficacy. In some respects, these terms speak for themselves. In-depth descriptions of these principles are provided in the resources listed in Table 4–5. The one principle that warrants additional elaboration is developing discrepancy. When people examine the

TABLE 4–8. **Motivational interviewing tools and exercises**

Strategy	Overview
1. Reviewing a typical day	Client discusses how substance use fits into his or her life, using an example of a typical day. Allows therapist to collect information and increase rapport.
2. Looking back	Client discusses life prior to substance use. Therapist uses OARS and assesses how the problematic behavior has changed over time. Goal is for client to perceive the immediacy of the circumstances, while perceiving change in behavior over time.
3. Decisional balance	Client identifies, then compares 1) "good things" and "not so good things" about changing drug use, as well as about 2) NOT changing. After client lists good and not so good things, therapist asks client an open question such as "What do you make of this?"
4. Discussing the stages of change	Therapist explains the stages of change and then follows up by asking for client's reaction, things client changed in the past, and examples of being in different stages of change.
5. Assessment feedback	Therapist provides formal or informal feedback about client's behavior. Therapist's role is to express this information, enabling the client to attribute meaning.
6. Values exploration	Therapist and client explore client's long-term and short-term values, allowing the client to define "ideal self." They can also explore consistency between values and behaviors, in addition to how problematic behaviors impact this consistency.
7. Looking forward	Client envisions two futures: 1) where he or she might be in 5–10 years if continuing same path without changes; 2) what that future might look like IF he or she decides to change behavior.

TABLE 4–8. Motivational interviewing tools and exercises *(continued)*

Strategy	Overview
8. Exploring importance and confidence (a.k.a. Rulers exercises)	Therapist and client explore client's perceptions of the importance of making a change, in addition to client's confidence in making a change. Client rates importance and confidence on a scale from 0 to 10. For low to mid-range ratings, therapist asks, "What makes you choose ___ [client's number] instead of ___ [some lower number]?"

Note. OARS=open-ended questions, affirming, reflective listening, and summarizing.
Source. Adapted from Ingersoll et al. 2000; Rosengren and Wagner 2001.

discrepancy between their current behavior and their values and goals, it can be overwhelming and generate negative affect. Well-trained therapists know that there is an optimal amount of arousal needed to motivate behavioral performance. Too low or too high arousal is associated with poor performance. Therefore, the strategies and communication style used by a provider need to be sensitive to the client's arousal level and not produce too much (as with heavy-handed approaches) or too little (as with a passive style). Also, with regard to avoiding arguing, it can sometimes be the case that providers are arguing without realizing that they are. The trick for the clinician is to learn to identify arguing and correct it in his or her practice.

Several exercises have been developed to facilitate conversation and provide some structure within which the OARS and the principles can be implemented. Table 4–8 presents a summary of these exercises. When you use these skills, there are some frequently encountered client responses. Table 4–9 provides examples of MI-consistent and -inconsistent responses to common client statements.

When a client's desire to quit is very strong but willpower and commitment to action are tentative, it can be helpful to start considering how to help the client cope with barriers to his or her self-efficacy and confidence. CBT-based techniques may be described or encouraged at this point while MI techniques are still being used. Interventions that teach actual skills are almost always required to help people with METH dependence. But how do you know when a client is ready for the next step in treatment and what potential barriers stand in the way? MI providers listen carefully for change talk—words clients use that indicate desire, reasons, need, and ability to change. When a client says anything in favor of change, the MI provider reflects those statements, affirms them, and elicits additional detail using open questions.

TABLE 4–9. Motivational interviewing: MI-consistent and -nonconsistent responses

Strategy	Client statement	Non-MI response	MI response
Decisional balance	1. I'm doing everything I'm supposed to do. I like doing it and it's my business.	1. There are consequences you are going to have to face.	1. As long as you aren't hurting anyone else, it doesn't make sense why people want you to stop.
	2. There is nothing good about using at all—nothing.	2. Well, why do you do it then?	2. The not so good things seem overwhelming to you. What made you keep using?
Looking back	1. I really had a rough childhood.	1. You have to let go of that. You can't let that keep being your excuse.	1. Drug use seemed almost unavoidable.
	2. If that friend hadn't kept pushing me, I never would have tried it.	2. You can't blame other people. The only person you can change is yourself.	2. It was hard to resist that pressure and you couldn't see a way to say no.
Looking forward	1. No one can predict how life is going to be.	1. If you don't start doing some planning, you're going to stay in this same boat.	1. Things may not go the way you want them to, so it isn't worth the effort to imagine a future.
	2. It's depressing to think about that.	2. This is hard work, but it's necessary.	2. It seems like it is going to be all bad and no good.

TABLE 4–9. Motivational interviewing: MI-consistent and -nonconsistent responses *(continued)*

Strategy	Client statement	Non-MI response	MI response
Exploring importance and confidence (a.k.a. Rulers exercises)	1. Importance is rated 9/10, and confidence is rated 2/10.	1. If you just stick with the program, you'll have what you need.	1. It's clear that changing is important to you. Tell me what it could take to make you more confident.
	2. Importance is rated 5/10, and confidence is rated 10/10.	2. Are you going to have to lose everything before this matters to you?	2. There is nothing at all that could get in your way if you decided this was important. What made you choose a 5 as opposed to a 3?

A message to keep in mind for very severe and chronically relapsing addiction is not to be tempted to give up on this approach if the client relapses. MI providers see ambivalence about changing behavior as expected and understand that progress still has been and may continue to be made even if relapse occurs. A pitfall that providers may fall into, especially regarding METH dependence, is to be overtaken by a sense of urgency and alarm that translates into more-confrontational behavior with clients that may result in client disengagement and defensiveness. It can be problematic to think of "getting the client to change" as the goal of MI. Therefore, it can be helpful to think of the goal of MI as to adhere to the MI style and skills and respond to change talk when it occurs and to focus on evoking and exploring ambivalence and reflecting what the client says about what makes him or her desire change.

To summarize, MI is used to decrease a person's ambivalence about changing his or her drug use and to increase the person's own internal desire for abstinence. MI skills are most obviously useful when working with a new client and/or a client who is not clearly verbalizing a strong commitment to change or desire for treatment. As such, MI sessions occur commonly before additional elements of an overall treatment program commence. However, MI skills can be integrated with other interventions, such as CM and CBT. There are no studies directly assessing the effectiveness of MI as a stand-alone intervention for METH dependence. MI is, however, an integral component of the community reinforcement approach (Budney and Higgins 1998). Its role in this approach is consistent with current evidence that suggests highly structured, long-term interventions are necessary for treatment efficacy for stimulant dependence.

KEY CLINICAL CONCEPTS

- Contingency management (CM) procedures require treatment providers to identify an appropriate target as well as an appropriate method for assessing the occurrence of the target behavior. Additionally, treatment providers must choose appropriate and effective reinforcers and decide the optimal way to deliver those reinforcers.

- Cognitive-behavioral therapy (CBT) for stimulant abuse includes functional analyses to determine the client's historic and current triggers for drug use, along with skills training in the management of drug cravings, effective drug-refusal techniques, and general problem-solving and decision-making strategies.

- Computerized delivery of CBT may effectively address issues commonly associated with regular in-person therapy sessions, such as scarcity of qualified mental health professionals in less populated regions, scheduling problems, transportation issues, and financial constraints.

- A variety of group counseling approaches exist, each with its own assumptions and approaches that can match the needs of a specific individual.

- Motivational interviewing (MI) is a technique used to decrease ambivalence about change and increase the person's own internal desire for abstinence.

- MI skills can be integrated with other interventions, such as CM and CBT.

- MI is not generally used as a stand-alone intervention; it is, however, an integral component of the community reinforcement approach.

Resources

Contingency Management

Higgins ST, Silverman S, Heil SH: Contingency Management in Substance Abuse Treatment. New York, Guilford, 2008
http://archives.drugabuse.gov/txmanuals/CRA/CRA1.html

Cognitive-Behavioral Therapy

Burns D: The Feeling Good Handbook. New York, Plume, 1999
Carroll KM: A Cognitive-Behavioral Approach: Treating Cocaine Addiction. Rockville, MD, National Institute on Drug Abuse, 1998
Center for Substance Abuse Treatment: Counselor's treatment manual: Matrix intensive outpatient treatment for people with stimulant use disorders (DHHS Publ No SMA-06-4152). 2006. Available at: http://www.oas.samhsa.gov/matrixStimulantHandbook/counselor.pdf. Accessed March 22, 2011.
Dobson D, Dobson KS: Evidence-Based Practice of Cognitive-Behavioral Therapy. New York, Guilford, 2009
Marlatt GA, Gordon JR (eds): Relapse Prevention. New York, Guilford, 1985
http://archives.drugabuse.gov/txmanuals/CBT/CBT1.html

Group Counseling

http://www.aa.org/
http://www.goodtherapy.org/Group-Therapy.html

References

Amrhein PC: How does motivational interviewing work? What client talk reveals. J Cogn Psychother 18:323–336, 2004

Amrhein PC, Miller WR, Yahne CE, et al: Client commitment language during motivational interviewing predicts drug use outcomes. J Consult Clin Psychol 71:862–878, 2003

Amrhein PC, Miller WR, Yahne C, et al: Strength of client commitment language improves with therapist training in motivational interviewing. Alcohol Clin Exp Res 28:74A, 2004

Amstadter AB, Broman-Fulks J, Zinzow H, et al: Internet-based interventions for traumatic stress-related mental health problems: a review and suggestion for future research. Clin Psychol Rev 29:410–420, 2009

Arkowitz H, Westra HA, Miller WR, et al (eds): Motivational Interviewing in the Treatment of Psychological Problems. New York, Guilford, 2008

Brehm JW: A Theory of Psychological Reactance. New York, Academic Press, 1966

Brehm SS, Brehm JW: Psychological Resistance: A Theory of Freedom and Control. New York, Academic Press, 1981

Bridle C, Riemsma RP, Pattenden J, et al: Systematic review of the effectiveness of health behavior interventions based on the transtheoretical model. Psychol Health 20:283–301, 2005

Budney AJ, Higgins ST: A Community Reinforcement Plus Vouchers Approach: Treating Cocaine Addiction. Washington, DC, National Institute on Drug Abuse, 1998

Carroll KM: A Cognitive-Behavioral Approach: Treating Cocaine Addiction. Rockville, MD, National Institute on Drug Abuse, 1998

Carroll KM, Fenton LR, Ball SA, et al: Efficacy of disulfiram and cognitive behavior therapy in cocaine-dependent outpatients: a randomized placebo-controlled trial. Arch Gen Psychiatry 61:264–272, 2004

Carroll KM, Ball SA, Martino S, et al: Computer-assisted delivery of cognitive-behavioral therapy for addiction: a randomized trial of CBT4CBT. Am J Psychiatry 165:881–888, 2008

Carroll KM, Ball SA, Martino S, et al: Enduring effects of a computer-assisted training program for cognitive behavioral therapy: a 6-month follow-up of CBT4CBT. Drug Alcohol Depend 100:178–181, 2009

Center for Substance Abuse Treatment: Counselor's treatment manual: matrix intensive outpatient treatment for people with stimulant use disorders. (DHHS Publ No SMA-06-4152). 2006. Available at: http://www.oas.samhsa.gov/matrixStimulantHandbook/counselor.pdf. Accessed March 22, 2011.

Cuijpers P, van Straten A, Andersson G: Internet-administered cognitive behavior therapy for health problems: a systematic review. J Behav Med 31:169–177, 2008

Dallery J, Glenn IM: Effects of an Internet-based voucher reinforcement program for smoking abstinence: a feasibility study. J Appl Behav Anal 38:349–357, 2005

Festinger L: A Theory of Cognitive Dissonance. Stanford, CA, Stanford University Press, 1957

Festinger L, Carlsmith JM: Cognitive consequences of forced compliance. J Abnorm Psychol 58:203–210, 1959

Garcia-Rodriguez O, Secades-Villa R, Higgins ST, et al: Financing a voucher program for cocaine abusers through community donations in Spain. J Appl Behav Anal 41:623–628, 2008

Higgins ST, Budney AJ, Bickel WK, et al: Achieving cocaine abstinence with a behavioral approach. Am J Psychiatry 150:763–769, 1993

Higgins ST, Badger GJ, Budney AJ: Initial abstinence and success in achieving longer term cocaine abstinence. Exp Clin Psychopharmacol 8:377–386, 2000

Ingersoll KS, Wagner CC, Gharib S: Motivational Groups for Community Substance Abuse Programs. Richmond, VA, Mid-Atlantic Addiction Technology Transfer Center, 2000

Kay-Lambkin FJ: Technology and innovation in the psychosocial treatment of methamphetamine use, risk and dependence. Drug Alcohol Rev 27:318–325, 2008

Lee NK, Rawson RA: A systematic review of cognitive and behavioural therapies for methamphetamine dependence. Drug Alcohol Rev 27:309–317, 2008

Litrell JH, Girvin H: Stages of change. A critique. Behav Modif 26:223–273, 2002

Lundahl B, Burke BL: The effectiveness and applicability of motivational interviewing: a practice-friendly review of four meta-analyses. J Clin Psychol 65:1232–1245, 2009

Lundahl BW, Kunz C, Brownell C, et al: A meta-analysis of motivational interviewing: twenty-five years of empirical studies. Res Soc Work Pract 20:137–160, 2010

Lussier JP, Heil SH, Mongeon JA, et al: A meta-analysis of voucher-based reinforcement therapy for substance use disorders. Addiction 101:192–203, 2006

Marlatt GA, Gordon JR (eds): Relapse Prevention. New York, Guilford, 1985

McHugh RK, Hearon BA, Otto MW: Cognitive behavioral therapy for substance use disorders. Psychiatr Clin North Am 33:511–525, 2010

Miller WR, Rollnick S: Motivational Interviewing: Preparing People for Change, 2nd Edition. New York, Guilford, 2002

Miller WR, Benefield RG, Tonigan JS: Enhancing motivation for change in problem drinking: a controlled comparison of two therapist styles. J Consult Clin Psychol 61:455–461, 1993

Penberthy JK, Ait-Daoud N, Vaughan M, et al: Review of treatment for cocaine dependence. Curr Drug Abuse Rev 3:49–62, 2010

Petry NM, Martin B: Low-cost contingency management for treating cocaine- and opioid-abusing methadone patients. J Consult Clin Psychol 70:398–405, 2002

Prochaska JO, DiClemente CC: The Transtheoretical Approach: Crossing Traditional Boundaries of Therapy. Homewood, IL, Dow Jones/Irwin, 1984

Prochaska JO, DiClemente CC, Norcross JC: In search of how people change: applications to addictive behaviors. Am Psychol 47:1102–1114, 1992

Project MATCH Research Group: Project MATCH secondary a priori hypotheses. Addiction 92:1671–1698, 1997

Rawson RA, Marinelli-Casey P, Anglin MD, et al: A multi-site comparison of psychosocial approaches for the treatment of methamphetamine dependence. Addiction 99:708–717, 2004

Roll JM, Higgins ST, Badger GJ: An experimental comparison of three different schedules of reinforcement of drug abstinence using cigarette smoking as an exemplar. J Appl Behav Anal 29:495–504; quiz 504–505, 1996

Rosengren D, Wagner CC: Motivational interviewing: dancing, not wrestling, in Addiction Recovery Tools: A Practitioner's Handbook. Edited by Coombs R. Thousand Oaks, CA, Sage, 2001, pp 17–34

Senay I, Albarracín D, Noguchi K: Motivating goal-directed behavior through introspective self-talk: the role of the interrogative form of simple future tense. Psychol Sci 21:499–504, 2010

Vernmark K, Lenndin J, Bjarehed J, et al: Internet administered guided self-help versus individualized e-mail therapy: a randomized trial of two versions of CBT for major depression. Behav Res Ther 48:368–376, 2010

Chapter 5

Pharmacotherapy

Thomas F. Newton, M.D.
Richard De La Garza II, Ph.D.
Ari D. Kalechstein, Ph.D.

Several practical and conceptual difficulties have slowed identification of effective medication treatments for stimulant dependence. The principal practical impediment has been that the pharmaceutical industry has not supported sufficient preclinical or clinical development. The principal conceptual problem is that researchers have not clearly defined what brain systems, and thus what neurotransmitter systems, should be targeted in order to help patients cut down or stop drug use. Because of these difficulties, earlier research was focused on treating syndromes thought to be linked to drug use, not on systems underpinning drug use. In this chapter, we review the rather extensive research literature describing the quest for a treatment for cocaine dependence and then close the chapter by reviewing the literature for the more recent quest for a treatment for methamphetamine (METH) dependence. Table 5–1 summarizes the potential medications for stimulant dependence that have been evaluated in clinical trials and other studies.

TABLE 5–1. Potential medications for stimulant dependence evaluated in clinical trials and other studies

Drug class	Medication	Primary drug target	Drug dependency	Overall efficacy (+/−)
Antidepressant	Desipramine	NE	Cocaine	−
	Fluoxetine	5-HT	Cocaine	−
	Bupropion	DA, NE	Cocaine, METH	−
	Gepirone	5-HT	Cocaine	−
	Venlafaxine	NE, 5-HT, DA	Cocaine	−
	Sertraline	5-HT	Cocaine	−
	Imipramine	NE, 5-HT	Cocaine	−
	Ritanserin	DA, 5-HT	Cocaine	−
Mood stabilizer/ Anticonvulsant	Carbamazepine	Sodium	Cocaine	−
	Lithium	Inositol triphosphate	Cocaine	−
	Phenytoin	Sodium, calcium	Cocaine	−
	Vigabatrin	GABA	Cocaine	+
	Tiagabine	GABA	Cocaine	+/−
	Baclofen	GABA	Cocaine	+/−
	Gabapentin	GABA	METH	+

TABLE 5–1. Potential medications for stimulant dependence evaluated in clinical trials and other studies *(continued)*

Drug class	Medication	Primary drug target	Drug dependency	Overall efficacy (+/−)
Dopamine agonist (indirect or direct)	Bromocriptine	DA	Cocaine, METH	+/−
	Pergolide	DA	Cocaine	−
	Amantadine	DA	Cocaine	
	Mazindol	DA	Cocaine	−
	Aripiprazole	DA	Cocaine, METH, AMPH	−
	Methylphenidate	DA	Cocaine, AMPH	+
	L-Dopa/Carbidopa	DA	Cocaine	+
	Modafinil	DA	Cocaine, METH	+
	SR-methamphetamine	DA	Cocaine	+
	SR-amphetamine	DA	Cocaine	+
Other				
Enzyme inhibitor	Disulfiram	DA, NE	Cocaine	
Antihypertensive	Nimodipine	Calcium	Cocaine	−

Note. 5-HT = serotonin; AMPH = amphetamine; DA = dopamine; GABA = γ-aminobutyric acid; METH = methamphetamine; NE = norepinephrine; SR = sustained-release.

Cocaine Dependence

Much effort has been expended evaluating antidepressants as potential treatments for cocaine dependence, beginning in the 1980s with the recognition of the devastation "crack" cocaine could cause. A promising human laboratory study suggested that desipramine, which acts primarily as a noradrenergic reuptake inhibitor, reduced cocaine-induced craving for cocaine (Fischman et al. 1990). An initial clinical trial suggested that desipramine might be an effective treatment (Gawin et al. 1989). Despite heroic efforts, subsequent research did not replicate this finding (Arndt et al. 1992; Campbell et al. 1994; Carroll et al. 1994; Feingold et al. 2002; Giannini et al. 1986, 1987; Hall et al. 1994; Kolar et al. 1992; Kosten et al. 1992; McElroy et al. 1989; O'Brien et al. 1988; Tennant and Tarver 1984; Triffleman et al. 1992; Weddington et al. 1991). Other antidepressants have been tested, based on similar rationales, including fluoxetine (Batki et al. 1993, 1996), bupropion (Margolin et al. 1995b), venlafaxine (McDowell et al. 2000), sertraline (Winhusen et al. 2005), and imipramine (Nunes et al. 1995). Thus far, none of these medications has proved effective for reducing cocaine use, at least when used alone (see discussion below on the effects of bupropion combined with contingency management).

Clinical trials of mood stabilizers, including carbamazepine (Brady et al. 2002; Campbell et al. 1994; Cornish et al. 1995; Halikas et al. 1997; Kranzler et al. 1995; Montoya et al. 1995) and lithium, have also been completed (Gawin et al. 1989), as have trials of phenytoin (Crosby et al. 1996) and direct or indirect dopamine agonists, including bromocriptine (Eiler et al. 1995; Giannini et al. 1989; Handelsman et al. 1997; Kranzler and Bauer 1992; Moscovitz et al. 1993; Tennant and Sagherian 1987), pergolide (Levin et al. 1999; Malcolm et al. 2000), amantadine (Alterman et al. 1992; Giannini et al. 1989; Handelsman et al. 1995; Kampman et al. 1996; Kolar et al. 1992; Kosten et al. 1992; Tennant and Sagherian 1987; Weddington et al. 1991), mazindol (Margolin et al. 1995a; Stine et al. 1995), and methylphenidate (Grabowski et al. 1997; Levin et al. 1998). A range of other agents, including ritanserin (Cornish et al. 2001; Johnson et al. 1997), gepirone (Jenkins et al. 1992), nimodipine (Rosse et al. 1994), and naltrexone (Oslin et al. 1999), have been studied as well. Aside from several weakly positive findings for modafinil (Anderson et al. 2009) and levodopa/carbidopa (Schmitz et al. 2008), none of these medications has proved reliably efficacious (Castells et al. 2007).

Studies of medications that were selected based on results of preclinical research have proved somewhat more promising. Vigabatrin is an inhibitor of γ-aminobutyric acid (GABA) transaminase, and inhibition of this enzyme results in greatly increased GABA levels. Brodie and colleagues showed that vigabatrin treatment reduced cocaine use in the final 2 weeks of their clinical trial (Brodie et al. 2009). Though these results are encouraging, vigabatrin can cause retinal abnormalities, and this will likely discourage use of this medication. Tiagabine inhibits the reuptake of GABA, and increases GABA levels, though not as potently as vigabatrin. Thus far, there have been mixed results, with one study finding benefit and one not (Gonzalez et al. 2003; Winhusen et al. 2007). Interestingly, the study that found that tiagabine helped patients reduce cocaine use included methadone-maintained patients (Gonzalez et al. 2003). Methadone maintenance increases retention and adherence, giving potentially effective medications a better chance to work. A similar finding was obtained for bupropion treatment during methadone maintenance coupled with contingency management treatment; the addition of bupropion reduced cocaine use. Contingency management offers incentives to patients (e.g., money) to stay in the study, thus ensuring the medication has a chance to act (Poling et al. 2006). Preclinical research suggests that baclofen, a $GABA_B$ agonist that reduces dopamine outflow from the ventral tegmental area, reduces cocaine-seeking behavior in rodents. An early clinical study suggested that baclofen may be effective for treating cocaine dependence (Shoptaw et al. 2003), although a subsequent study did not replicate this finding (Kahn et al. 2009).

Another potentially helpful medication was discovered more or less serendipitously. Reasoning that alcohol may facilitate relapse in cocaine users attempting to abstain from cocaine, several researchers identified disulfiram, a treatment for alcoholism, as a potential treatment for cocaine dependence. Several clinical trials then showed that disulfiram treatment reduced cocaine use, and surprisingly, this effect was independent of concomitant alcohol use (Carroll et al. 2000, 2004; George et al. 2000; Higgins et al. 1993; Petrakis et al. 2000). It was subsequently discovered that disulfiram inhibits many enzymes in addition to aldehyde dehydrogenase (the basis for its efficacy for alcoholism), including dopamine β-hydroxylase, the enzyme that is responsible for the synthesis of norepinephrine from dopamine. Unfortunately, disulfiram also inhibits the esterases responsible for the degradation of cocaine, so that repeated cocaine use during disulfiram treatment results in cocaine accumulation, with consequent high plasma levels (McCance-Katz et al. 1998). In studies to date, this effect has not led to adverse reactions, but it is concerning nonetheless.

A second approach, the so-called agonist treatment approach, is based on the reasoning that since the most effective treatment for opiate abuse is therapeutic treatment with a long-acting alternative opiate—for example, with methadone—stimulant substitution might effectively treat cocaine abuse. Several relatively small clinical trials of amphetamine (AMPH) and METH for cocaine dependence suggested that extended-release METH may prove to be both safe and effective for reducing cocaine use in selected users (Grabowski et al. 2001, 2004; Mooney et al. 2009). Several preclinical studies in rats and monkeys conducted in parallel with this line of research confirmed that AMPH treatment reduces the reinforcing effects of cocaine, but only after several days of treatment (Chiodo et al. 2008; Negus 2003; Negus and Mello 2003). A recent human laboratory study confirmed that AMPH treatment reduces the positive subjective effects of cocaine without enhancing aversive stimulant side effects such as anxiety (Rush et al. 2009). This is consistent with the preclinical research, as positive subjective effects frequently parallel reinforcing effects (Fischman 1989). There are obvious practical difficulties associated with using high-abuse-potential medications like AMPHs in patients with cocaine dependence, though these findings do provide provocative evidence that similar medications having less abuse potential may be useful.

More recently, investigators have used human laboratory studies to identify medications that reduce the reinforcing effects of cocaine, with the idea that this would identify effective treatments. This approach attempts to model real-world cocaine use while participants are in the laboratory, by allowing cocaine-dependent volunteers to choose between receiving cocaine or experiencing some other contingency, which might be positive (receiving money) or not (completing a work requirement or losing money). Several medications reduced the positive subjective effects of experimentally administered cocaine without reducing reinforcing effects, measured using self-administration procedures (Haney et al. 1998; Hart et al. 2004; Walsh et al. 2001), and some reduced both the subjective and reinforcing effects of cocaine (Hart et al. 2008), but thus far these studies have not led to the identification of an effective treatment. Nevertheless, this approach is necessary to determine the safety of putative treatments and remains the most face-valid method for identifying treatments.

Methamphetamine Dependence

There are fewer studies examining potential medication treatments for METH dependence. In one of the first studies published, participants received baclofen, gabapentin, or placebo (Heinzerling et al. 2006). Gabapentin was ineffective, but there was some evidence that baclofen reduced METH use in those who were highly adherent to the prescribed treatment (i.e., the interaction between number of pills reportedly taken and treatment group was significantly associated with urine drug screen results). In a subsequent study, bupropion pretreatment reduced the positive subjective effects of METH administered in the laboratory, and in two subsequent clinical trials, bupropion treatment was associated with reduced METH use in participants reporting relatively light use, but not in those reporting heavier use. More recently, a study from Finland found that slow-release methylphenidate was effective for reducing AMPH use, whereas patients receiving aripiprazole showed increased use (Tiihonen et al. 2007). The latter finding with aripiprazole is consistent with a published human laboratory study showing that aripiprazole pretreatment enhanced some of the abuse-related effects produced by METH (Newton et al. 2008). Finally, a study in Australia found that there was a trend for reduced METH use among treatment-adherent patients who were receiving modafinil (Shearer et al. 2009).

KEY CLINICAL CONCEPTS

- Cost of drug development and lack of interest by the pharmaceutical industry have been impediments in finding new drugs for stimulant dependence.

- Researchers have not been able to define precisely what neurobiological targets will produce therapeutically efficacious effects.

- Studies testing antidepressants have largely been negative, with the exception of bupropion, which decreases METH use in light users but not heavy users.

- Medications that increase GABA levels, such as vigabatrin and tiagabine, reduce cocaine use but have side effects that preclude their use. Baclofen has also been shown to decrease METH use.

- Numerous clinical studies show that disulfiram decreases cocaine use independent of alcohol use. Disulfiram, however, blocks enzymes that metabolize cocaine, thereby increasing peripheral levels, which could be detrimental.

- Promising studies using an agonist treatment approach showed that sustained-release formulations of AMPH, METH, and methylphenidate used to treat attention-deficit/hyperactivity disorder block the subjective effects and decrease cocaine use. Methylphenidate has also shown positive effects for amphetamine dependence. Abuse liability precludes these compounds from being used clinically, however.

- Positive clinical studies continue to support modafinil as a possible pharmacotherapy for cocaine and METH dependence.

Resources

Journal Article

Ross S, Peselow E: Pharmacotherapy of addictive disorders. Clin Neuropharmacol 32, 277–289, 2009

Website

National Institute on Drug Abuse: The Science of Addiction
http://www.nida.nih.gov/DrugPages/addiction.html

References

Alterman AI, Droba M, Antelo RE, et al: Amantadine may facilitate detoxification of cocaine addicts. Drug Alcohol Depend 31:19–29, 1992

Anderson AL, Reid MS, Li SH, et al: Modafinil for the treatment of cocaine dependence. Drug Alcohol Depend 104:133–139, 2009

Arndt IO, Dorozynsky L, Woody GE, et al: Desipramine treatment of cocaine dependence in methadone-maintained patients. Arch Gen Psychiatry 49:888–893, 1992

Batki SL, Manfredi LB, Jacob PD, et al: Fluoxetine for cocaine dependence in methadone maintenance: quantitative plasma and urine cocaine/benzoylecgonine concentrations. J Clin Psychopharmacol 13:243–250, 1993

Batki SL, Washburn AM, Delucchi K, et al: A controlled trial of fluoxetine in crack cocaine dependence. Drug Alcohol Depend 41:137–142, 1996

Brady KT, Sonne SC, Malcolm RJ, et al: Carbamazepine in the treatment of cocaine dependence: subtyping by affective disorder. Exp Clin Psychopharmacol 10:276–285, 2002

Brodie JD, Case BG, Figueroa E, et al: Randomized, double-blind, placebo-controlled trial of vigabatrin for the treatment of cocaine dependence in Mexican parolees. Am J Psychiatry 166:1269–1277, 2009

Campbell JL, Thomas HM, Gabrielli W, et al: Impact of desipramine or carbamazepine on patient retention in outpatient cocaine treatment: preliminary findings. J Addict Dis 13:191–199, 1994

Carroll KM, Rounsaville BJ, Gordon LT, et al: Psychotherapy and pharmacotherapy for ambulatory cocaine abusers. Arch Gen Psychiatry 51:177–187, 1994

Carroll KM, Nich C, Ball SA, et al: One-year follow-up of disulfiram and psychotherapy for cocaine-alcohol users: sustained effects of treatment. Addiction 95:1335–1349, 2000

Carroll KM, Fenton LR, Ball SA, et al: Efficacy of disulfiram and cognitive behavior therapy in cocaine-dependent outpatients: a randomized placebo-controlled trial. Arch Gen Psychiatry 61:264–272, 2004

Castells X, Casas M, Vidal X, et al: Efficacy of central nervous system stimulant treatment for cocaine dependence: a systematic review and meta-analysis of randomized controlled clinical trials. Addiction 102:1871–1887, 2007. doi:10.1111/j.1360-0443.2007.01943

Chiodo KA, Lack CM, Roberts DC: Cocaine self-administration reinforced on a progressive ratio schedule decreases with continuous D-amphetamine treatment in rats. Psychopharmacology (Berl) 200:465–473, 2008

Cornish JW, Maany I, Fudala PJ, et al: Carbamazepine treatment for cocaine dependence. Drug Alcohol Depend 38:221–227, 1995

Cornish JW, Maany I, Fudala PJ, et al: A randomized, double-blind, placebo-controlled study of ritanserin pharmacotherapy for cocaine dependence. Drug Alcohol Depend 61:183–189, 2001

Crosby RD, Pearson VL, Eller C, et al: Phenytoin in the treatment of cocaine abuse: a double-blind study. Clin Pharmacol Ther 59:458–468, 1996

de Lima MS, de Oliveira Soares BG, Reisser AA, et al: Pharmacological treatment of cocaine dependence: a systematic review. Addiction 97:931–949, 2002

Eiler K, Schaefer MD, Salstrom D, et al: Double-blind comparison of bromocriptine and placebo in cocaine withdrawal. Am J Drug Alcohol Abuse 21:65–79, 1995

Feingold A, Oliveto A, Schottenfeld R, et al: Utility of crossover designs in clinical trials: efficacy of desipramine vs. placebo in opioid-dependent cocaine abusers. Am J Addict 11:111–123, 2002

Fischman MW: Relationship between self-reported drug effects and their reinforcing effects: studies with stimulant drugs. NIDA Res Monogr 92:211–230, 1989

Fischman MW, Foltin RW, Nestadt G, et al: Effects of desipramine maintenance on cocaine self-administration by humans. J Pharmacol Exp Ther 253:760–770, 1990

Gawin FH, Kleber HD, Byck R, et al: Desipramine facilitation of initial cocaine abstinence. Arch Gen Psychiatry 46:117–121, 1989

George TP, Chawarski MC, Pakes J, et al: Disulfiram versus placebo for cocaine dependence in buprenorphine-maintained subjects: a preliminary trial. Biol Psychiatry 47:1080–1086, 2000

Giannini AJ, Malone DA, Giannini MC, et al: Treatment of depression in chronic cocaine and phencyclidine abuse with desipramine. J Clin Pharmacol 26:211–214, 1986

Giannini AJ, Loiselle RH, Giannini MC: Space-based abstinence: alleviation of withdrawal symptoms in combinative cocaine-phencyclidine abuse. J Toxicol Clin Toxicol 25:493–500, 1987

Giannini AJ, Folts DJ, Feather JN, et al: Bromocriptine and amantadine in cocaine detoxification. Psychiatry Res 29:11–16, 1989

Gonzalez G, Sevarino K, Sofuoglu M, et al: Tiagabine increases cocaine-free urines in cocaine-dependent methadone-treated patients: results of a randomized pilot study. Addiction 98:1625–1632, 2003

Grabowski J, Roache JD, Schmitz JM, et al: Replacement medication for cocaine dependence: methylphenidate. J Clin Psychopharmacol 17:485–488, 1997

Grabowski J, Rhoades H, Schmitz J, et al: Dextroamphetamine for cocaine-dependence treatment: a double-blind randomized clinical trial. J Clin Psychopharmacol 21:522–526, 2001

Grabowski J, Rhoades H, Stotts A, et al: Agonist-like or antagonist-like treatment for cocaine dependence with methadone for heroin dependence: two double-blind randomized clinical trials. Neuropsychopharmacology 29:969–981, 2004

Halikas JA, Crosby RD, Pearson VL, et al: A randomized double-blind study of carbamazepine in the treatment of cocaine abuse. Clin Pharmacol Ther 62:89–105, 1997

Hall SM, Tunis S, Triffleman E, et al: Continuity of care and desipramine in primary cocaine abusers. J Nerv Ment Dis 182:570–575, 1994

Handelsman L, Limpitlaw L, Williams D, et al: Amantadine does not reduce cocaine use or craving in cocaine-dependent methadone maintenance patients. Drug Alcohol Depend 39:173–180, 1995

Handelsman L, Rosenblum A, Palij M, et al: Bromocriptine for cocaine dependence: a controlled clinical trial. Am J Addict 6:54–64, 1997

Haney M, Foltin RW, Fischman MW: Effects of pergolide on intravenous cocaine self-administration in men and women. Psychopharmacology (Berl) 137:15–24, 1998

Hart CL, Ward AS, Collins ED, et al: Gabapentin maintenance decreases smoked cocaine-related subjective effects, but not self-administration by humans. Drug Alcohol Depend 73:279–287, 2004

Hart CL, Haney M, Vosburg SK, et al: Smoked cocaine self-administration is decreased by modafinil. Neuropsychopharmacology 33:761–768, 2008

Heinzerling KG, Shoptaw S, Peck JA, et al: Randomized, placebo-controlled trial of baclofen and gabapentin for the treatment of methamphetamine dependence. Drug Alcohol Depend 85:177–184, 2006

Higgins ST, Budney AJ, Bickel WK, et al: Disulfiram therapy in patients abusing cocaine and alcohol. Am J Psychiatry 150:675–676, 1993

Jenkins SW, Warfield NA, Blaine JD, et al: A pilot trial of gepirone vs. placebo in the treatment of cocaine dependency. Psychopharmacol Bull 28:21–26, 1992

Johnson BA, Chen YR, Swann AC, et al: Ritanserin in the treatment of cocaine dependence. Biol Psychiatry 42:932–940, 1997

Kahn R, Biswas K, Childress AR, et al: Multi-center trial of baclofen for abstinence initiation in severe cocaine-dependent individuals. Drug Alcohol Depend 103:59–64, 2009

Kampman K, Volpicelli JR, Alterman A, et al: Amantadine in the early treatment of cocaine dependence: a double-blind, placebo-controlled trial. Drug Alcohol Depend 41:25–33, 1996

Kolar AF, Brown BS, Weddington WW, et al: Treatment of cocaine dependence in methadone maintenance clients: a pilot study comparing the efficacy of desipramine and amantadine. Int J Addict 27:849–868, 1992

Kosten TR, Morgan CM, Falcione J, et al: Pharmacotherapy for cocaine-abusing methadone-maintained patients using amantadine or desipramine. Arch Gen Psychiatry 49:894–898, 1992

Kranzler HR, Bauer LO: Bromocriptine and cocaine cue reactivity in cocaine-dependent patients. Br J Addict 87:1537–1548, 1992

Kranzler HR, Bauer LO, Hersh D, et al: Carbamazepine treatment of cocaine dependence: a placebo-controlled trial. Drug Alcohol Depend 38:203–211, 1995

Levin FR, Evans SM, McDowell DM, et al: Methylphenidate treatment for cocaine abusers with adult attention-deficit/hyperactivity disorder: a pilot study. J Clin Psychiatry 59:300–305, 1998

Levin FR, McDowell D, Evans SM, et al: Pergolide mesylate for cocaine abuse: a controlled preliminary trial. Am J Addict 8:120–127, 1999

Malcolm R, Kajdasz DK, Herron J, et al: A double-blind, placebo-controlled outpatient trial of pergolide for cocaine dependence. Drug Alcohol Depend 60:161–168, 2000

Margolin A, Avants SK, Kosten TR: Mazindol for relapse prevention to cocaine abuse in methadone-maintained patients. Am J Drug Alcohol Abuse 21:469–481, 1995a

Margolin A, Kosten TR, Avants SK, et al: A multicenter trial of bupropion for cocaine dependence in methadone-maintained patients. Drug Alcohol Depend 40:125–131, 1995b

McCance-Katz EF, Kosten TR, Jatlow P: Chronic disulfiram treatment effects on intranasal cocaine administration: initial results. Biol Psychiatry 43:540–543, 1998

McDowell DM, Levin FR, Seracini AM, et al: Venlafaxine treatment of cocaine abusers with depressive disorders. Am J Drug Alcohol Abuse 26:25–31, 2000

McElroy SL, Weiss RD, Mendelson JH, et al: Desipramine treatment for relapse prevention in cocaine dependence. NIDA Res Monogr 95:57–63, 1989

Montoya ID, Levin FR, Fudala PJ, et al: Double-blind comparison of carbamazepine and placebo for treatment of cocaine dependence. Drug Alcohol Depend 38:213–219, 1995

Mooney ME, Herin DV, Schmitz JM, et al: Effects of oral methamphetamine on cocaine use: a randomized, double-blind, placebo-controlled trial. Drug Alcohol Depend 101:34–41, 2009

Moscovitz H, Brookoff D, Nelson L: A randomized trial of bromocriptine for cocaine users presenting to the emergency department. J Gen Intern Med 8:1–4, 1993

Negus SS: Rapid assessment of choice between cocaine and food in rhesus monkeys: effects of environmental manipulations and treatment with d-amphetamine and flupenthixol. Neuropsychopharmacology 28:919–931, 2003

Negus SS, Mello NK: Effects of chronic d-amphetamine treatment on cocaine- and food-maintained responding under a second-order schedule in rhesus monkeys. Drug Alcohol Depend 70:39–52, 2003

Newton TF, Reid MS, De La Garza R, et al: Evaluation of subjective effects of aripiprazole and methamphetamine in methamphetamine-dependent volunteers. Int J Neuropsychopharmacol 11:1037–1045, 2008

Nunes EV, McGrath PJ, Quitkin FM, et al: Imipramine treatment of cocaine abuse: possible boundaries of efficacy. Drug Alcohol Depend 39:185–195, 1995

O'Brien CP, Childress AR, Arndt IO, et al: Pharmacological and behavioral treatments of cocaine dependence: controlled studies. J Clin Psychiatry 49(suppl):17–22, 1988

Oslin DW, Pettinati HM, Volpicelli JR, et al: The effects of naltrexone on alcohol and cocaine use in dually addicted patients. J Subst Abuse Treat 16:163–167, 1999

Petrakis IL, Carroll KM, Nich C, et al: Disulfiram treatment for cocaine dependence in methadone-maintained opioid addicts. Addiction 95:219–228, 2000

Poling J, Oliveto A, Petry N, et al: Six-month trial of bupropion with contingency management for cocaine dependence in a methadone-maintained population. Arch Gen Psychiatry 63:219–228, 2006

Rosse RB, Alim TN, Fay-McCarthy M, et al: Nimodipine pharmacotherapeutic adjuvant therapy for inpatient treatment of cocaine dependence. Clin Neuropharmacol 17:348–358, 1994

Rush CR, Stoops WW, Hays LR: Cocaine effects during D-amphetamine maintenance: a human laboratory analysis of safety, tolerability and efficacy. Drug Alcohol Depend 99:261–271, 2009

Schmitz JM, Mooney ME, Moeller FG, et al: Levodopa pharmacotherapy for cocaine dependence: choosing the optimal behavioral therapy platform. Drug Alcohol Depend 94:142–150, 2008

Shearer J, Darke S, Rodgers C, et al: A double-blind, placebo-controlled trial of modafinil (200 mg/day) for methamphetamine dependence. Addiction 104:224–233, 2009

Shoptaw S, Yang X, Rotheram-Fuller EJ, et al: Randomized placebo-controlled trial of baclofen for cocaine dependence: preliminary effects for individuals with chronic patterns of cocaine use. J Clin Psychiatry 64:1440–1448, 2003

Stine SM, Krystal JH, Kosten TR, et al: Mazindol treatment for cocaine dependence. Drug Alcohol Depend 39:245–252, 1995

Tennant FS Jr, Sagherian AA: Double-blind comparison of amantadine and bromocriptine for ambulatory withdrawal from cocaine dependence. Arch Intern Med 147:109–112, 1987

Tennant FS Jr, Tarver AL: Double-blind comparison of desipramine and placebo in withdrawal from cocaine dependence. NIDA Res Monogr 55:159–163, 1984

Tiihonen J, Kuoppasalmi K, Fohr J, et al: A comparison of aripiprazole, methylphenidate, and placebo for amphetamine dependence. Am J Psychiatry 164:160–162, 2007

Triffleman E, Delucchi K, Tunis S, et al: Desipramine in the treatment of "crack" cocaine dependence. Preliminary results. NIDA Monograph Series 132:317, 1992

Walsh SL, Geter-Douglas B, Strain EC, et al: Enadoline and butorphanol: evaluation of kappa-agonists on cocaine pharmacodynamics and cocaine self-administration in humans. J Pharmacol Exp Ther 299:147–158, 2001

Weddington WW Jr, Brown BS, Haertzen CA, et al: Comparison of amantadine and desipramine combined with psychotherapy for treatment of cocaine dependence. Am J Drug Alcohol Abuse 17:137–152, 1991

Winhusen TM, Somoza EC, Harrer JM, et al: A placebo-controlled screening trial of tiagabine, sertraline and donepezil as cocaine dependence treatments. Addiction 100 (suppl 1):68–77, 2005

Winhusen T[M], Somoza E, Ciraulo DA, et al: A double-blind, placebo-controlled trial of tiagabine for the treatment of cocaine dependence. Drug Alcohol Depend 91:141–148, 2007

Chapter 6

Polydrug Abuse

Richard De La Garza II, Ph.D.
Ari D. Kalechstein, Ph.D.

As discussed in earlier chapters, the use of cocaine or methamphetamine (METH) is associated with long-term changes to a number of neurotransmitter and second messenger systems and is accompanied by significant deleterious effects on the health of the individual. While thousands of studies have examined the independent effects of cocaine, METH, nicotine, marijuana, alcohol, and opiates on the human brain and behavior, fewer studies have examined the effects of the combined use of these substances. This lack of research is unfortunate, since any knowledgeable health care provider or researcher who has encountered cocaine- or METH-dependent individuals knows that polydrug use is the norm. Finding a patient who abuses only cocaine or only METH is atypical. Most stimulant users use these drugs in combination, often with the intent either to increase the effects produced by the primary stimulant or to "take the edge off" a high when they want to control the cardiovascular and subjective effects.

The principal concern of polydrug use is that relative to the use of a single drug, the additive effects of multiple drugs create an increased risk for the onset of adverse consequences, such as cardiovascular toxicity or neurocognitive impairment. In addition, it is not known to what extent abuse of other substances compromises or complicates treatment outcomes. While it has been known for years that these other addictive drugs activate many of the same brain regions and neurotransmitter systems implicated in cocaine and METH dependence, the most exciting development involves new data showing that there is shared genetic risk for dependence on multiple substances (Kendler et al. 2007; Sherva et al. 2010). In this chapter, we summarize some of the key findings that have been put forth on the topic of concurrent use of stimulants and other drugs, highlighting nicotine, marijuana, alcohol, and opiates, since they are the most commonly abused substances.

Stimulants and Nicotine

Subjective Effects

A number of studies have examined the combined subjective effects of nicotine and cocaine in individuals dependent on cocaine. In an early report, Roll and colleagues (1997) conducted a study with healthy volunteers under controlled laboratory conditions. Participants received double-blind doses of intranasal cocaine or placebo in separate sessions, followed by a 3-hour period of monitored cigarette smoking. Latency to the first cigarette and the mean interval between cigarettes were significantly shorter, and the total number of cigarettes smoked was greater, after cocaine exposure than after placebo exposure. In the same report, urine specimens were collected from ambulatory cocaine-dependent patients. Urine cotinine (a primary metabolite of nicotine) levels were significantly higher on days that patients tested positive for cocaine use, indicating that cocaine use was associated with increased cigarette smoking. Overall, these results indicate that cocaine use can increase cigarette smoking. These data do not, however, match outcomes of a study in which computerized cigarette dispensers were used to evaluate the effects of multiple daily cocaine administrations on cigarette smoking (Radzius et al. 1997). In this report, participants resided on a closed clinical research ward and 3 days per week could obtain either cocaine or saline. The investigators reported no change in the number of cigarettes smoked after chronic cocaine self-administration. These data are in line with outcomes of a study in which increased cocaine effect was perceived by only 15% of simultaneous cigarette users (Wiseman and McMillan 1996), implying that additive effects are uncommon among cocaine users.

Several laboratory studies have been conducted in an attempt to advance our understanding of the effects produced by nicotine in cocaine-dependent users. In one study, the subjective and physiological effects of intravenously administered cocaine and nicotine were compared in 10 cigarette-smoking cocaine abusers (Jones et al. 1999). Under double-blind conditions, subjects received placebo, cocaine, or nicotine in randomized fashion. Nicotine showed a more rapid onset of subjective effects than cocaine, and both drugs increased subjective ratings of "drug effect," "rush," "good effects," "liking," "high," and "stimulated," while nicotine alone increased ratings of "bad effects" and "jittery." Interestingly, the highest nicotine dose produced greater effects than the highest cocaine dose on most subjective measures. Notwithstanding, at doses that produced comparable ratings of drug effect, cocaine produced significantly greater good effects, whereas nicotine produced greater bad effects. Also of interest, high nicotine doses were frequently categorized as producing effects similar to those of cocaine or amphetamine. In a second study, volunteers were first treated with a transdermal nicotine patch (14 mg) and then challenged with an acute dose of intranasal cocaine (Kouri et al. 2001). The data showed that nicotine pretreatment attenuated cocaine-induced increases in "high" and "stimulated," and increased the latency to detect cocaine effects and cocaine-induced euphoria. In contrast, another study revealed that transdermal nicotine (21 mg) maintenance did not alter increases in subjective and reinforcing effects produced by intravenous cocaine (Sobel et al. 2004). To confuse matters, a recent study showed that the positive subjective effects ("high" and "rush") produced by intravenous cocaine began to decrease within one or two puffs of a high-nicotine cigarette while nicotine levels were increasing (Mello 2010). Taken together, the available data are mixed, with some studies showing increases, one showing no change, and one showing that nicotine reduces the subjective effects produced by cocaine.

To our knowledge, there are no comparable laboratory studies evaluating the combined subjective effects produced by METH and nicotine in humans.

Physiological Effects

Several studies have examined the combined cardiovascular effects of nicotine in individuals dependent on cocaine. Cocaine-related cardiovascular complications include acute myocardial ischemia and infarction, arrhythmias, sudden death, myocarditis, cardiomyopathy, hypertension, aortic ruptures, and endocarditis. In one review, development of a cocaine-related cardiovascular event was described as being potentiated by concurrent use of nicotine and other substances (Maraj et al. 2010). In the study mentioned earlier in the context of subjective effects, nicotine and cocaine increased blood pressure and heart rate and decreased skin temperature in cigarette-smoking cocaine abusers (Jones et al. 1999), and the magnitude of changes was similar for these drugs in a side-by-side comparison. In the study by Lukas and colleagues (Kouri et al. 2001), pretreatment with transdermal nicotine did not alter cocaine's effects on heart rate, skin temperature, and blood pressure. This outcome is similar to the study conducted by Griffiths and

colleagues (Sobel et al. 2004) in which intravenous cocaine produced significant elevations in heart rate and blood pressure, though no consistent effects
of pretreatment with transdermal nicotine were observed. Again, as observed
with subjective effects, the available data are conflicting, with some reports
showing increases and others showing decreases produced by combined nicotine and cocaine exposure.

Few studies have evaluated the effects of nicotine use in METH-dependent
individuals. In one study, lifetime use and recent use of nicotine did not predict cardiovascular responses to METH administered in the laboratory (Fleury
et al. 2008).

Treatment Outcomes

According to a recent review, early exposure to nicotine influences the development of stimulant addiction, and smokers with comorbid drug use
have more severe stimulant use and may be more treatment resistant (Weinberger and Sofuoglu 2009). A reasonable concern among treatment providers is that successful reduction of cocaine use might be accompanied by
increased tobacco smoking. This concern appears unfounded given outcomes in a trial of 168 crack cocaine–dependent patients entering a 12-week
outpatient treatment program (Patkar et al. 2006). As expected, cocaine-
dependent patients improved with treatment and showed significant reduction in scores on the Addiction Severity Index, yet there were no significant
changes in number of cigarettes smoked per day or scores on the Fagerström
Test for Nicotine Dependence (FTND) from baseline to end of treatment or
follow-up. In an earlier study of 43 cocaine users, patients reported significant reductions in cigarette consumption after cessation of cocaine use, and
this effect was most pronounced among heavy smokers (Wiseman and Mc-
Millan 1998).

Given the known overlap of effects of cocaine, METH, and nicotine on
neurotransmitter systems, it is not surprising that some of the most effective
medications for smoking cessation have also been evaluated specifically for
treating stimulant dependence. In theory, if the medications prove effective
for both addictive disorders, then much will have been gained by using one
medication instead of two. For example, the first-line treatment for nicotine
dependence, varenicline, is being evaluated for cocaine dependence (Crunelle et al. 2010; Guillem and Peoples 2010; Poling et al. 2010) and for
METH dependence (Zorick et al. 2009). Another example includes bupropion, which remains an effective treatment option for smoking cessation and
has been evaluated for cocaine dependence (Levin et al. 2002; Oliveto et al.
2001; Poling et al. 2006; Shoptaw et al. 2008a) and for METH dependence
(Elkashef et al. 2008; Newton et al. 2006; Shoptaw et al. 2008b). Importantly,

modafinil appears to be a good candidate medication for cocaine dependence (Dackis et al. 2003; Hart et al. 2008; Martinez-Raga et al. 2008; Volkow et al. 2009) and perhaps METH dependence (De La Garza et al. 2010; Kalechstein et al. 2010) but has been shown to accentuate cigarette smoking (Schnoll et al. 2008). Similarly, topiramate has been considered for cocaine dependence (Reis et al. 2008), but one report showed that topiramate enhanced the subjective effects produced by nicotine, indicating that individuals receiving this medication might be compelled to smoke cigarettes more often (Sofuoglu et al. 2006). This finding was supported by a study showing that topiramate treatment enhanced the rewarding effects of a smoked cigarette (Reid et al. 2007). These latter examples serve as a cautionary note for clinicians, who must take into consideration smoking behavior in their patients.

Of interest to our research group and others are acetylcholinesterase inhibitors, which increase acetylcholine in the brain in a manner similar to that of nicotine, as potential treatments for cocaine dependence. So far the data are equivocal: one report showed potential efficacy (Grasing et al. 2010) and the only other showed that donepezil was not better than placebo (Winhusen et al. 2005). Notwithstanding, the known interactions between the acetylcholine and dopamine systems in the brain highlight the fact that drugs that directly or indirectly target acetylcholine levels warrant careful consideration as treatments for cocaine dependence (Williams and Adinoff 2008).

A recent report indicates that nicotine dependence can be used as a predictor of adherence to treatment for METH dependence (Dean et al. 2009). Specifically, the authors reported that infrequent METH abusers with low FTND scores were highly likely to drop out of treatment (88% dropping out), while infrequent users with higher FTND scores were more likely to remain in treatment (30% dropping out). Our research group has shown that the acetylcholinesterase inhibitor rivastigmine significantly reduced "desire for methamphetamine" among METH-dependent individuals (De La Garza et al. 2008). These data highlight the potential usefulness of drugs that target acetylcholine systems as treatments for METH dependence.

Stimulants and Cannabis

Subjective Effects

In one study, research volunteers received intravenous cocaine and smoked cannabis alone and in combination during daily experimental sessions (Foltin et al. 1993). The data show that both cocaine alone and cannabis alone increased ratings of "stimulated" and "high," and there was a trend for combinations of these drugs to prolong these elevations.

Physiological Effects

Current use of cannabis was negatively correlated with peak heart rate change after acute METH exposure in the laboratory, and male cannabis users showed lower peak change in heart rate as compared with non–cannabis users (Fleury et al. 2008). Among cocaine users, combinations of intravenous cocaine and smoked cannabis increased heart rate over and above levels seen with either drug alone (Foltin et al. 1995). In a separate study, adult male research volunteers received cocaine and cannabis, alone and in combination, during experimental sessions (Foltin and Fischman 1990). The combination of cocaine and cannabis produced increases in heart rate that were similar to those seen with cannabis alone. The same group had earlier conducted an even more telling laboratory experiment, in which intravenous cocaine was administered after the start of cannabis smoking (a 1-gram marijuana cigarette) (Foltin et al. 1987). Cocaine alone produced dose-dependent increases in heart rate, while both low and high tetrahydrocannabinol (THC) blood levels produced a similar increase in heart rate. Both doses of cocaine increased mean arterial pressure similarly, while THC alone produced blood level–dependent increases in mean arterial pressure. Combinations of cocaine and cannabis increased heart rate above levels seen with either drug alone.

Neurocognition

In a recent study, Cunha et al. (2010) compared neurocognitive function in 30 substance-dependent individuals and 32 healthy individuals, using a Frontal Assessment Battery and other executive control function tasks. Substance-dependent individuals demonstrated poorer performance than control subjects in three of the six cognitive domains. Interestingly, some neuropsychological measures were correlated with the amount of alcohol, cannabis, and cocaine use. In another study, nondependent stimulant users performed markedly less well in comparison to stimulant-naive subjects on the learning, free recall, and recognition portions of the California Verbal Learning Test, 2nd Edition (CVLT-II). Interestingly, lifetime use of stimulants and cannabis did not affect performance on the CVLT-II (Reske et al. 2010). These findings are consistent with those from a study comparing cocaine-free polydrug control subjects and cocaine polydrug users matched for sex, age, alcohol consumption, and IQ (Colzato et al. 2009). The results show that cocaine polydrug users (who had monthly cannabis use rates four times greater than those of the cocaine-free control subjects) exhibited reduced attentional function. This finding, the authors speculated, may be associated with the perpetuation of the use of the drug and may explain why it is so difficult for cocaine users to change their compulsive drug-related habits and to enter and stay in rehabilitation therapy.

Treatment Outcomes

Lindsay et al. (2009) evaluated cannabis use in 1,183 individuals seeking outpatient treatment for cocaine dependence. The data reveal that cocaine-dependent patients with frequent cannabis intake used more cocaine and alcohol and reported more medical, legal, and psychiatric problems, including antisocial personality disorder. These data have important and obvious treatment implications. Notwithstanding, these findings appear at odds with findings from a study that investigated the effects of cannabis use on treatment retention and abstinence from cocaine among cocaine-dependent patients with attention-deficit/hyperactivity disorder (ADHD) (Aharonovich et al. 2006). Cocaine-dependent patients diagnosed with current ADHD participated in a randomized clinical trial of methylphenidate for treatment of ADHD and cocaine dependence in an outpatient setting. The majority of patients (69%) used cannabis during treatment. Surprisingly, the analyses revealed that increased cannabis use was associated with greater treatment retention.

According to recent reviews, the endocannabinoid system might not only block the direct reinforcing effect of cannabis, opioids, nicotine, and ethanol, but also prevent the relapse to various drugs of abuse, including opioids, cocaine, nicotine, alcohol, and amphetamine (Parolaro and Rubino 2008; Tanda 2007). Cannabinoid-1 (CB1) antagonists are obvious choices as medications for marijuana dependence (Huestis et al. 2007) and are also being considered for cocaine and METH dependence, though trials with the CB1 antagonist rimonabant have not been conducted in humans and will not likely occur because of U.S. Food and Drug Administration safety concerns. Other CB1 antagonists are being developed, and only time will tell whether these compounds have applications outside of marijuana dependence.

There are other factors to consider in assessing the impact of cannabis use in stimulant-dependent individuals, including the concern that cannabis use may produce and/or exacerbate psychotic symptoms in vulnerable individuals. In one study, cannabis-use history was obtained from 1,140 cocaine-dependent individuals (Kalayasiri et al. 2010). The results showed that cocaine-dependent individuals who endorsed cocaine-induced psychosis had significantly higher rates of adolescent-onset cannabis use compared with those who did not report cocaine-induced psychosis. These findings are distinct from those of a study showing that age at onset of psychosis treatment was significantly associated with the use of cannabis, but independent of the use of cocaine, tobacco smoking, or excessive alcohol consumption (Barrigón et al. 2010).

Stimulants and Alcohol

Subjective Effects

A number of double-blind, placebo-controlled laboratory-based studies have examined the independent and combined effects of cocaine and alcohol on subjective response in individuals dependent on cocaine and alcohol. Initial studies showed that the concurrent administration of cocaine and alcohol resulted in greater euphorigenic effects than those produced by cocaine alone (e.g., Foltin and Fischman 1988; Harris et al. 2003; McCance-Katz et al. 1993, 1998). Examples of euphorigenic effects included self-reported "high" and "feels good." Moreover, these studies showed that the combination of cocaine and alcohol resulted in the production of cocaethylene as measured in urine (Harris et al. 2003) and in plasma (McCance-Katz et al. 1993, 1998), and that the level of cocaethylene in plasma was positively associated with the dose of cocaine administered (Harris et al. 2003). Another study showed subtle gender effects, such that women showed greater perceptions of well-being relative to men at equivalent doses (McCance-Katz et al. 2005). It was suggested that this difference in perception was related to an indication that, in general, women require more time to metabolize cocaethylene than men.

To our knowledge, one study has examined the degree to which alcohol modulates the effects of METH (Mendelson et al. 1995). In that double-blind placebo-controlled study, participants reported that "subjective intoxication" was greater subsequent to the combined administration of METH and alcohol than it was after the solo administration of METH or alcohol. No other subjective effects were reported.

Physiological Effects

Variable findings have been observed in studies that examined the manner in which alcohol influences physiological responses to cocaine. Three studies found that the combination of cocaine and alcohol was associated with markedly increased heart rate relative to cocaine and placebo, but differences were not observed with respect to systolic and diastolic blood pressure (Foltin and Fischman 1988; McCance-Katz et al. 1993, 1998). In contrast, another study showed that the administration of cocaine and alcohol was associated with notable increases in heart rate, systolic blood pressure, and diastolic blood pressure (McCance-Katz et al. 2005); in this study, gender did not moderate the combined effects of cocaine and alcohol versus cocaine on cardiovascular functioning.

In the double-blind placebo-controlled study that examined the degree to which alcohol modulates the physiological effects of METH (Mendelson et al. 1995, discussed above), systolic blood pressure and heart rate were lower subsequent to the combined administration of METH and alcohol than they were after the solo administration of METH or alcohol. Diastolic blood pressure was lower as well, though the result did not meet the threshold for significance.

Neuroimaging

A literature search using PubMed yielded two studies that investigated the differential effect of alcohol on brain imaging in samples of recently abstinent cocaine-dependent individuals. One study utilized structural neuroimaging to examine the relative effects of alcohol in a sample of individuals who had been abstinent for 16–18 weeks, on average (O'Neill et al. 2001). In that report, individuals dependent on cocaine and alcohol had lower prefrontal white matter volumes, particularly in the area of the anterior cingulate, relative to individuals using either cocaine or alcohol, but not both. The other study involving cocaine-dependent individuals examined cerebral blood flow in participants who had been abstinent from alcohol for at least 24 hours, and 26 of the 32 participants had not used cocaine for at least 96 hours prior to undergoing the brain scan (Gottschalk and Kosten 2002). The analyses revealed that cocaine- and alcohol-dependent individuals showed greater levels of hypoperfusion in the temporal and occipital cortices or the cerebellum, and greater levels of hypoperfusion in the frontal and parietal cortices, relative to cocaine-only users.

To our knowledge, one study, using magnetic resonance imaging, has examined whether alcohol use mediates the results of structural neuroimaging in amphetamine-dependent individuals (Lawyer et al. 2010). The study preliminarily suggested that heavy alcohol use exacerbates the deleterious effects of alcohol, such that the patient group exhibited reduced cortical thickness in the superior-frontal right hemisphere and the precentral left hemisphere.

Neurocognition

A literature search using PubMed yielded three studies that investigated the differential effect of alcohol on neurocognition in samples of recently abstinent cocaine-dependent individuals. (There were no studies that examined this effect in samples of METH-dependent individuals.) For example, one study evaluated participants within 1–3 days of abstinence initiation and then repeated the evaluation after 4 weeks of abstinence (Bolla et al. 2000). The study authors reported that the combined detrimental effects of cocaine and alcohol on measures of attention/information processing speed, learning and memory, and executive functioning were greater than the independent effects of cocaine and alcohol. The findings reported by Bolla and colleagues contrasted with those from other studies. For instance, one study, which evaluated study participants who had been abstinent for 72 hours, reported that with respect to mean ratings of global neurocognitive impairment on measures of attention, motoric function, and information processing speed, individuals using cocaine and alcohol and those using cocaine alone performed similarly to matched control subjects (Robinson et al. 1999). Moreover, in that same study, the prevalence of impaired performance was greater in cocaine users relative to matched control subjects and individuals using cocaine and alcohol. Similar findings were obtained in a sample of individuals who had been abstinent for 1–14 days, particularly on measures of memory (Abi-Saab et al. 2005).

Three more studies evaluated the relative effects of cocaine and alcohol on neurocognition following longer periods of abstinence, ranging from approximately 6 to 52 weeks (Di Sclafani et al. 1998, 2002; Lawton-Craddock et al. 2003). Each of the studies consistently showed that alcohol use generally did not modulate the effects of cocaine on neurocognitive functioning, indexed as mean performance on tests for each group. However, one of the studies showed that increased intracranial volume was associated with a reduced likelihood of the onset of neurocognitive impairment (Di Sclafani et al. 1998). Another showed higher peak doses of alcohol and cocaine and higher amounts of average use were risk factors for onset of impairment, as indexed by global scores of neurocognitive functioning (Di Sclafani et al. 2002).

Treatment Outcomes

A series of studies have examined the relative influence of alcohol with respect to cocaine-addicted individuals' capacity to remain abstinent following admission to treatment. In contrast, we did not identify studies that examined the manner in which opiate use influenced treatment outcomes in cocaine-dependent individuals. Moreover, to our knowledge, no studies have examined the relative efficacy of pharmacological and/or psychosocial treatments in samples of METH-dependent individuals with/without alcohol or opiate dependence.

A subset of the studies examined the efficacy of behavioral treatments in cocaine-dependent individuals who were or were not alcohol dependent. One study found that individuals addicted to cocaine and alcohol were more likely to use cocaine prior to and immediately following outpatient relapse prevention treatment, though the group differences were minimal at the 12- and 24-week follow-up assessments (Schmitz et al. 1997). Another study examined the efficacy of contingency management over a 9-month period in groups of cocaine users, a subset of whom also were cocaine dependent (Rash et al. 2008). In this study, alcohol use did not influence treatment outcomes. In contrast, a study involving nonspecific behavioral treatment reported that individuals abusing cocaine and alcohol were more likely to be depressed and/or psychotic, more likely to show poorer overall functioning, and less likely to attend treatment sessions than were individuals abusing cocaine (Brady et al. 1995). Similar findings were obtained in a 26-week study, which showed that alcohol use at the 4-week mark of the study was associated with reduced likelihood of maintaining abstinence from cocaine (Mengis et al. 2002).

Other studies examined the degree to which candidate medications influenced treatment outcomes. In one study, pergolide administration did not modulate cocaine or alcohol use, indexed as clean urine toxicology screens, in cocaine-dependent individuals with or without co-occurring alcohol dependence (Malcolm et al. 2000). In contrast, disulfiram administration was associated with reduced cocaine use in cocaine-dependent individuals, particularly in the subset of study participants who were not dependent on alcohol at the time of study entry and those participants who abstained from alcohol during the study (Carroll et al. 2004). Similar findings were obtained in a 12-week outpatient study examining the relative efficacy of modafinil (Anderson et al. 2009), such that administration of the medication was associated with a greater proportion of days remaining abstinent in individuals without a history of alcohol dependence.

Some studies examined the relative influence of alcohol without recruiting separate groups of substance users (i.e., cocaine users who were or were not dependent on alcohol). The results of these studies have been mixed (for review, see Poling et al. 2007). For example, one study showed that alcohol use variables, such as alcohol use, alcohol craving, and alcohol withdrawal symptoms, were not related to whether participants successfully completed outpatient detoxification (Kampman et al. 2004), whereas another study yielded dissimilar findings (McKay et al. 1999). A third study showed that history of alcohol use generally was unrelated to abstinence from cocaine, measured by urine toxicology screens and self-report (Ahmadi et al. 2006). Finally, an epidemiological study with a sample size in excess of 36,000 participants showed that concurrent use of alcohol and cocaine was associated with an array of negative outcomes, including increased psychiatric comorbidity, increased use of cigarettes and marijuana, and greater likelihood of arrest, relative to cocaine use only (Hedden et al. 2009).

Stimulants and Opiates

Subjective Effects

To our knowledge, no studies have examined the manner in which heroin influences subjective responses to cocaine or METH; however, one study examined the incremental effects of hydromorphone on the subjective effects of cocaine administration (Walsh et al. 1996). In that study, concurrent administration of cocaine and hydromorphone was associated with an increased "drug effect" relative to cocaine or hydromorphone alone, but did not affect "high," "euphoria," or "stimulated."

Other studies utilized a different methodology, in which the effects of cocaine were evaluated in opiate-addicted individuals who were being maintained on methadone, buprenorphine, or some other heroin substitute. One study showed that cocaine administration was associated with significant increases in "high," "stimulated," and "good drug effect," and that the effect did not differ across methadone or buprenorphine (Foltin and Fischman 1996). Moreover, in a sample of methadone-maintained addicts, the effects of cocaine were evident regardless of whether the cocaine was administered 1 hour or 22 hours after the dose of methadone (Foltin et al. 1995).

Physiological Effects

To our knowledge, only one study has examined the incremental effects of an opiate—in this case, hydromorphone—on the physiological effects produced by cocaine administration (Walsh et al. 1996). In this report, concurrent administration of cocaine and hydromorphone was associated with increased systolic and diastolic blood pressure, increased heart rate, and reduced pupil diameter. For studies of the incremental effects of cocaine on the physiological functioning of methadone-maintained addicts, relatively similar findings were obtained—namely, cocaine was associated with increased stress on the cardiovascular system. This finding occurred regardless of whether single or multiple doses of cocaine were administered (Foltin et al. 1995), whether the cocaine was administered 1 hour or 22 hours after the dose of methadone (Foltin et al. 1995), or whether cocaine was administered in the context of methadone or buprenorphine (Foltin and Fischman 1996). A more recent study examined the relative effects of cocaine and nalbuphine on the hypothalamic-pituitary-adrenal axis (Goletiani et al. 2009). The study showed that administration of nalbuphine reduced serum adrenocorticotropic hormone, cortisol, and luteinizing hormone following cocaine administration.

Treatment Outcomes

To our knowledge, no studies have examined the incremental effects of opiate use on treatment outcomes for individuals primarily addicted to stimulants. This is not surprising, as the studies in this area have recruited participants who are primarily addicted to opiates and who may or may not also be addicted to stimulants.

Conclusion

In this chapter, we considered use of one stimulant plus one other drug, when in fact we know that the vast majority of individuals are using multiple substances at any given time. Considering all possible combinations is beyond the scope of this review. Nonetheless, the information provided in this chapter clearly illustrates the challenges and confounds that polydrug abuse may have on treatment outcomes for stimulant-dependent individuals.

KEY CLINICAL CONCEPTS

- Most stimulant-dependent individuals also use, or are dependent on, another drug of abuse, such as nicotine, cannabis, alcohol, or opiates. These drugs alter the positive subjective effects of stimulants and may increase the incidence of adverse events.

- *Nicotine* dependence is present in a high percentage of stimulant-dependent individuals. Nicotine affects cocaine's positive and negative subjective effects and increases the likelihood of adverse cardiovascular events.

- Individuals dependent on nicotine and cocaine may be more resistant to treatment.

- Because common neurobiological mechanisms are shared between nicotine and cocaine, medications for smoking cessation are being tested for treatment of cocaine and methamphetamine dependence.

- Drugs that show promise for treatment of cocaine dependence, such as modafinil and topiramate, enhance the subjective effects of nicotine.

- *Cannabis* enhances cocaine's subjective and physiological effects and may trigger psychosis in vulnerable individuals.

- Many neurocognitive parameters are affected by simultaneous use of cannabis and cocaine.

- *Alcohol* enhances cocaine's subjective effects, and this may be a function of the metabolite cocaethylene. Alcohol also enhances some of methamphetamine's subjective effects.

- Alcohol increases cocaine's physiological effects, whereas it decreases the effects produced by methamphetamine.

- Imaging studies show alcohol enhances the deleterious effects of cocaine on specific brain structures in addition to impairing cognitive and motor function.

- Disulfiram, a medication used to treat alcohol dependence, decreases cocaine use regardless of alcohol drinking status. In contrast, modafinil does not decrease cocaine use in individuals with a history of alcohol dependence.

- *Opiates* increase cocaine's subjective and physiological effects.

Resources

http://www.drugabuse.gov/NIDA_notes/NNvol22N1/New.html
Surhone LM, Timpledon MT, Marseken SF (eds): Poly Drug Use. Betascript Publishing, 2010

References

Abi-Saab D, Beauvais J, Mehm J, et al: The effect of alcohol on the neuropsychological functioning of recently abstinent cocaine-dependent subjects. Am J Addict 14:166–178, 2005

Aharonovich E, Garawi F, Bisaga A, et al: Concurrent cannabis use during treatment for comorbid ADHD and cocaine dependence: effects on outcome. Am J Drug Alcohol Abuse 32:629–635, 2006

Ahmadi J, Kampman K, Dackis C: Outcome predictors in cocaine dependence treatment trials. Am J Addict 15:434–439, 2006

Anderson AL, Reid MS, Li SH, et al: Modafinil for the treatment of cocaine dependence. Drug Alcohol Depend 104:133–139, 2009

Barrigón ML, Gurpegui M, Ruiz-Veguilla M, et al: Temporal relationship of first-episode non-affective psychosis with cannabis use: a clinical verification of an epidemiological hypothesis. J Psychiatr Res 44:413–420, 2010

Bolla KI, Funderburk F, Cadet JL: Differential effects of cocaine and cocaine + alcohol on neurocognitive performance. Neurology 54:2285–2292, 2000

Brady KT, Sonne S, Randall CL, et al: Features of cocaine dependence with concurrent alcohol abuse. Drug Alcohol Depend 39:69–71, 1995

Carroll KM, Fenton LR, Ball SA, et al: Efficacy of disulfiram and cognitive behavior therapy in cocaine-dependent outpatients: a randomized placebo-controlled trial. Arch Gen Psychiatry 61:264–272, 2004

Colzato LS, Huizinga M, Hommel B: Recreational cocaine polydrug use impairs cognitive flexibility but not working memory. Psychopharmacology (Berl) 207:225–234, 2009

Crunelle CL, Miller ML, Booij J, et al: The nicotinic acetylcholine receptor partial agonist varenicline and the treatment of drug dependence: a review. Eur Neuropsychopharmacol 20:69–79, 2010

Cunha PJ, Nicastri S, de Andrade AG, et al: The Frontal Assessment Battery (FAB) reveals neurocognitive dysfunction in substance-dependent individuals in distinct executive domains: abstract reasoning, motor programming, and cognitive flexibility. Addict Behav 35:875–881, 2010

Dackis CA, Lynch KG, Yu E, et al: Modafinil and cocaine: a double-blind, placebo-controlled drug interaction study. Drug Alcohol Depend 70:29–37, 2003

Dean AC, London ED, Sugar CA, et al: Predicting adherence to treatment for methamphetamine dependence from neuropsychological and drug use variables. Drug Alcohol Depend 105:48–55, 2009

De La Garza R [2nd], Shoptaw S, Newton TF: Evaluation of the cardiovascular and subjective effects of rivastigmine in combination with methamphetamine in methamphetamine-dependent human volunteers. Int J Neuropsychopharmacol 11:729–741, 2008

De La Garza R 2nd, Zorick T, London ED, et al: Evaluation of modafinil effects on cardiovascular, subjective, and reinforcing effects of methamphetamine in methamphetamine-dependent volunteers. Drug Alcohol Depend 106:173–180, 2010

Di Sclafani V, Clark HW, Tolou-Shams M, et al: Premorbid brain size is a determinant of functional reserve in abstinent crack-cocaine and crack-cocaine-alcohol-dependent adults. J Int Neuropsychol Soc 4:559–565, 1998

Di Sclafani V, Tolou-Shams M, Price LJ, et al: Neuropsychological performance of individuals dependent on crack-cocaine, or crack-cocaine and alcohol, at 6 weeks and 6 months of abstinence. Drug Alcohol Depend 66:161–171, 2002

Elkashef AM, Rawson RA, Anderson AL, et al: Bupropion for the treatment of methamphetamine dependence. Neuropsychopharmacology 33:1162–1170, 2008

Fleury G, De La Garza R 2nd, Mahoney JJ 3rd, et al: Predictors of cardiovascular response to methamphetamine administration in methamphetamine-dependent individuals. Am J Addict 17:103–110, 2008

Foltin RW, Fischman MW: Ethanol and cocaine interactions in humans: cardiovascular consequences. Pharmacol Biochem Behav 31:877–883, 1988

Foltin RW, Fischman MW: The effects of combinations of intranasal cocaine, smoked marijuana, and task performance on heart rate and blood pressure. Pharmacol Biochem Behav 36:311–315, 1990

Foltin RW, Fischman MW: Effects of methadone or buprenorphine maintenance on the subjective and reinforcing effects of intravenous cocaine in humans. J Pharmacol Exp Ther 278:1153–1164, 1996

Foltin RW, Fischman MW, Pedroso JJ, et al: Marijuana and cocaine interactions in humans: cardiovascular consequences. Pharmacol Biochem Behav 28:459–464, 1987

Foltin RW, Fischman MW, Pippen PA, et al: Behavioral effects of cocaine alone and in combination with ethanol or marijuana in humans. Drug Alcohol Depend 32:93–106, 1993

Foltin RW, Christiansen I, Levin FR, et al: Effects of single and multiple intravenous cocaine injections in humans maintained on methadone. J Pharmacol Exp Ther 275:38–47, 1995

Goletiani NV, Mendelson JH, Sholar MB, et al: Opioid and cocaine combined effect on cocaine-induced changes in HPA and HPG axes hormones in men. Pharmacol Biochem Behav 91:526–536, 2009

Gottschalk PC, Kosten TR: Cerebral perfusion defects in combined cocaine and alcohol dependence. Drug Alcohol Depend 68:95–104, 2002

Grasing K, Mathur D, Newton TF, et al: Donepezil treatment and the subjective effects of intravenous cocaine in dependent individuals. Drug Alcohol Depend 107:69–75, 2010

Guillem K, Peoples LL: Varenicline effects on cocaine self administration and reinstatement behavior. Behav Pharmacol 21:96–103, 2010

Harris DS, Everhart ET, Mendelson J, et al: The pharmacology of cocaethylene in humans following cocaine and ethanol administration. Drug Alcohol Depend 72:169–182, 2003

Hart CL, Haney M, Vosburg SK, et al: Smoked cocaine self-administration is decreased by modafinil. Neuropsychopharmacology 33:761–768, 2008

Hedden SL, Malcolm RJ, Latimer WW: Differences between adult non-drug users versus alcohol, cocaine and concurrent alcohol and cocaine problem users. Addict Behav 34:323–326, 2009

Huestis MA, Boyd SJ, Heishman SJ, et al: Single and multiple doses of rimonabant antagonize acute effects of smoked cannabis in male cannabis users. Psychopharmacology (Berl) 194:505–515, 2007

Jones HE, Garrett BE, Griffiths RR: Subjective and physiological effects of intravenous nicotine and cocaine in cigarette smoking cocaine abusers. J Pharmacol Exp Ther 288:188–197, 1999

Kalayasiri R, Gelernter J, Farrer L, et al: Adolescent cannabis use increases risk for cocaine-induced paranoia. Drug Alcohol Depend 107:196–201, 2010

Kalechstein AD, De La Garza R 2nd, Newton TF: Modafinil administration improves working memory in methamphetamine-dependent individuals who demonstrate baseline impairment. Am J Addict 19:340–344, 2010

Kampman KM, Pettinati HM, Volpicelli JR, et al: Cocaine dependence severity predicts outcome in outpatient detoxification from cocaine and alcohol. Am J Addict 13:74–82, 2004

Kendler KS, Myers J, Prescott CA: Specificity of genetic and environmental risk factors for symptoms of cannabis, cocaine, alcohol, caffeine, and nicotine dependence. Arch Gen Psychiatry 64:1313–1320, 2007

Kouri EM, Stull M, Lukas SE: Nicotine alters some of cocaine's subjective effects in the absence of physiological or pharmacokinetic changes. Pharmacol Biochem Behav 69:209–217, 2001

Lawton-Craddock A, Nixon SJ, Tivis R: Cognitive efficiency in stimulant abusers with and without alcohol dependence. Alcohol Clin Exp Res 27:457–464, 2003

Lawyer G, Bjerkan PS, Hammarberg A, et al: Amphetamine dependence and comorbid alcohol abuse: associations to brain cortical thickness. BMC Pharmacol 10:5, 2010

Levin FR, Evans SM, McDowell DM, et al: Bupropion treatment for cocaine abuse and adult attention-deficit/hyperactivity disorder. J Addict Dis 21:1–16, 2002

Lindsay JA, Stotts AL, Green CE, et al: Cocaine dependence and concurrent marijuana use: a comparison of clinical characteristics. Am J Drug Alcohol Abuse 35:193–198, 2009

Malcolm R, Kajdasz DK, Herron J, et al: A double-blind, placebo-controlled outpatient trial of pergolide for cocaine dependence. Drug Alcohol Depend 60:161–168, 2000

Maraj S, Figueredo VM, Lynn Morris D: Cocaine and the heart. Clin Cardiol 33:264–269, 2010

Martinez-Raga J, Knecht C, Cepeda S: Modafinil: a useful medication for cocaine addiction? Review of the evidence from neuropharmacological, experimental and clinical studies. Curr Drug Abuse Rev 1:213–221, 2008

McCance-Katz EF, Price LH, McDougle CJ, et al: Concurrent cocaine-ethanol ingestion in humans: pharmacology, physiology, behavior, and the role of cocaethylene. Psychopharmacology (Berl) 111:39–46, 1993

McCance-Katz EF, Kosten TR, Jatlow P: Concurrent use of cocaine and alcohol is more potent and potentially more toxic than use of either alone—a multiple-dose study. Biol Psychiatry 44:250–259, 1998

McCance-Katz EF, Hart CL, Boyarsky B, et al: Gender effects following repeated administration of cocaine and alcohol in humans. Subst Use Misuse 40:511–528, 2005

McKay JR, Alterman AI, Rutherford MJ, et al: The relationship of alcohol use to cocaine relapse in cocaine dependent patients in an aftercare study. J Stud Alcohol 60:176–180, 1999

Mello NK: Hormones, nicotine, and cocaine: clinical studies. Horm Behav 58:57–71, 2010

Mendelson J, Jones RT, Upton R, et al: Methamphetamine and ethanol interactions in humans. Clin Pharmacol Ther 57:559–568, 1995

Mengis MM, Maude-Griffin PM, Delucchi K, et al: Alcohol use affects the outcome of treatment for cocaine abuse. Am J Addict 11:219–227, 2002

Newton TF, Roache JD, De La Garza R 2nd, et al: Bupropion reduces methamphetamine-induced subjective effects and cue-induced craving. Neuropsychopharmacology 31:1537–1544, 2006

Oliveto A, McCance-Katz FE, Singha A, et al: Effects of cocaine prior to and during bupropion maintenance in cocaine-abusing volunteers. Drug Alcohol Depend 63:155–167, 2001

O'Neill J, Cardenas VA, Meyerhoff DJ: Separate and interactive effects of cocaine and alcohol dependence on brain structures and metabolites: quantitative MRI and proton MR spectroscopic imaging. Addict Biol 6:347–361, 2001

Parolaro D, Rubino T: The role of the endogenous cannabinoid system in drug addiction. Drug News Perspect 3:149–157, 2008

Patkar AA, Mannelli P, Peindl K, et al: Changes in tobacco smoking following treatment for cocaine dependence. Am J Drug Alcohol Abuse 32:135–148, 2006

Poling J, Oliveto A, Petry N, et al: Six-month trial of bupropion with contingency management for cocaine dependence in a methadone-maintained population. Arch Gen Psychiatry 63:219–228, 2006

Poling J, Kosten TR, Sofuoglu M: Treatment outcome predictors for cocaine dependence. Am J Drug Alcohol Abuse 33:191–206, 2007

Poling J, Rounsaville B, Gonsai K, et al: The safety and efficacy of varenicline in cocaine using smokers maintained on methadone: a pilot study. Am J Addict 19:401–408, 2010

Radzius A, Carriero NJ, Weinhold LL, et al: Changes in cigarette smoking not observed following repeated cocaine self-administration. Exp Clin Psychopharmacol 5:51–53, 1997

Rash CJ, Alessi SM, Petry NM: Cocaine abusers with and without alcohol dependence respond equally well to contingency management treatments. Exp Clin Psychopharmacol 16:275–281, 2008

Reid MS, Palamar J, Raghavan S, et al: Effects of topiramate on cue-induced cigarette craving and the response to a smoked cigarette in briefly abstinent smokers. Psychopharmacology (Berl) 192:147–158, 2007

Reis AD, Castro LA, Faria R, et al: Craving decrease with topiramate in outpatient treatment for cocaine dependence: an open label trial. Rev Bras Psiquiatr 30:132–135, 2008

Reske M, Eidt CA, Delis DC, et al: Nondependent stimulant users of cocaine and prescription amphetamines show verbal learning and memory deficits. Biol Psychiatry 68:762–769, 2010

Robinson JE, Heaton RK, O'Malley SS: Neuropsychological functioning in cocaine abusers with and without alcohol dependence. J Int Neuropsychol Soc 5:10–19, 1999

Roll JM, Higgins ST, Tidey J: Cocaine use can increase cigarette smoking: evidence from laboratory and naturalistic settings. Exp Clin Psychopharmacol 5:263–268, 1997

Schmitz JM, Bordnick PS, Kearney ML, et al: Treatment outcome of cocaine-alcohol dependent patients. Drug Alcohol Depend 47:55–61, 1997

Schnoll RA, Wileyto EP, Pinto A, et al: A placebo-controlled trial of modafinil for nicotine dependence. Drug Alcohol Depend 98:86–93, 2008

Sherva R, Kranzler HR, Yu Y, et al: Variation in nicotinic acetylcholine receptor genes is associated with multiple substance dependence phenotypes. Neuropsychopharmacology 35:1921–1931, 2010

Shoptaw S, Heinzerling KG, Rotheram-Fuller E, et al: Bupropion hydrochloride versus placebo, in combination with cognitive behavioral therapy, for the treatment of cocaine abuse/dependence. J Addict Dis 27:13–23, 2008a

Shoptaw S, Heinzerling KG, Rotheram-Fuller E, et al: Randomized, placebo-controlled trial of bupropion for the treatment of methamphetamine dependence. Drug Alcohol Depend 96:222–232, 2008b

Sobel BF, Sigmon SC, Griffiths RR: Transdermal nicotine maintenance attenuates the subjective and reinforcing effects of intravenous nicotine, but not cocaine or caffeine, in cigarette-smoking stimulant abusers. Neuropsychopharmacology 29:991–1003, 2004

Sofuoglu M, Poling J, Mouratidis M, et al: Effects of topiramate in combination with intravenous nicotine in overnight abstinent smokers. Psychopharmacology (Berl) 184:645–651, 2006

Tanda G: Modulation of the endocannabinoid system: therapeutic potential against cocaine dependence. Pharmacol Res 56:406–417, 2007

Volkow ND, Fowler JS, Logan J, et al: Effects of modafinil on dopamine and dopamine transporters in the male human brain: clinical implications. JAMA 301:1148–1154, 2009

Walsh SL, Sullivan JT, Preston KL, et al: Effects of naltrexone on response to intravenous cocaine, hydromorphone and their combination in humans. J Pharmacol Exp Ther 279:524–538, 1996

Weinberger AH, Sofuoglu M: The impact of cigarette smoking on stimulant addiction. Am J Drug Alcohol Abuse 35:12–17, 2009

Williams MJ, Adinoff B: The role of acetylcholine in cocaine addiction. Neuropsychopharmacology 33:1779–1797, 2008

Winhusen TM, Somoza EC, Harrer JM, et al: A placebo-controlled screening trial of tiagabine, sertraline and donepezil as cocaine dependence treatments. Addiction 100 (suppl 1):68–77, 2005

Wiseman EJ, McMillan DE: Combined use of cocaine with alcohol or cigarettes. Am J Drug Alcohol Abuse 22:577–587, 1996

Wiseman EJ, McMillan DE: Relationship of cessation of cocaine use to cigarette smoking in cocaine-dependent outpatients. Am J Drug Alcohol Abuse 24:617–625, 1998

Zorick T, Sevak RJ, Miotto K, et al: Pilot safety evaluation of varenicline for the treatment of methamphetamine dependence. J Exp Pharmacol 2010:13–18, 2009

Chapter 7

HIV and Other Medical Comorbidity

Valerie A. Gruber, Ph.D., M.P.H.
Elinore F. McCance-Katz, M.D., Ph.D.

Although most of the time people use cocaine or methamphetamine (METH) without noticing any negative health consequences, serious medical problems can occur, sometimes suddenly and sometimes insidiously. Studies of cocaine- or METH-related deaths in coroners' information systems (Graham and Hanzlick 2008; Kaye et al. 2008) showed that stimulants were rated as the direct cause of death in 25% of cocaine-related deaths and 73% of METH-related deaths, causing an adverse event such as a brain hemorrhage in 20% of cocaine-related deaths and 11% of METH-related deaths, or complicating other disease in 55% of cocaine-related deaths and 16% of METH-related deaths. In this chapter, we review research on the most common medical consequences of cocaine and METH use, including overdose, cumulative effects on various organ systems, behavior changes resulting in injuries, and infectious diseases. Understanding these effects may be helpful in motivating stimulant users to stop harmful patterns of use. With regard to individuals' chronic medical conditions brought on by stimulant use, we discuss how stimulant use affects the medical management of these conditions, with a focus on HIV.

Effects of Cocaine and Methamphetamine on the Body

Stimulant Overdose

METH overdose can result in multiple organ failure resembling heatstroke, including shock, convulsions, and coma (Lan et al. 1998). Individuals in cocaine or METH overdose present initially with symptoms such as agitation, tremor, increased heart rate and temperature, and excited delirium (for review, see Darke et al. 2008). Children of stimulant users, especially infants, may be accidentally exposed via dust or smoke; early symptoms of METH toxicity in children include tachycardia, vomiting, irritability, and hyperactivity (McGuinness and Pollack 2008). Following prolonged stimulant exposure, hyperthermia and dehydration can cause muscle breakdown (rhabdomyolysis) and kidney failure (e.g., Richards et al. 1999; Ruttenber et al. 1999) if not immediately treated. Stimulant-using patients with sudden back pain not related to an injury should be evaluated for possible renal toxicity. Because stimulant use can be associated with sudden death, it is helpful for staff working with stimulant users to be trained in basic life support/cardiopulmonary resuscitation.

Cardiovascular System

Cocaine use increases risk of myocardial infarction and sudden cardiac death via a combination of mechanisms, including hypertension, vasoconstriction, vasospasm, thrombus (blood clot) formation, arrhythmia, and aortic dissection (rupture) (for reviews, see Phillips et al. 2009 [cocaine] and Kaye et al. 2007 [METH]). Individuals with preexisting structural cardiac disease, including cardiomyopathy or atherosclerosis, are at higher risk. In a study of U.S. emergency department (ED) admissions for decompensated heart failure, stimulant users (96% cocaine users, 4% METH users) were younger and more likely to be African American (Diercks et al. 2008). In a study of HIV-positive patients without cardiovascular symptoms, cocaine use for over 15 years more than doubled the odds of coronary stenosis, even after other factors, such as antiretroviral treatment, were controlled for (Lai et al. 2008). Combined cocaine and cigarette smoking has been shown to synergistically decrease diameters of diseased segments of coronary arteries, with diameters decreasing 9% with cocaine, 5% with smoking, and 19% with cocaine and smoking (Moliterno et al. 1994). Vasoconstriction is also the likely mechanism for the association of METH use with retinal artery occlusion and corneal ulcers/scarring with resulting vision defects or loss (Hazin et al. 2009).

Bill, a 46-year-old man, had symptomatic HIV (CD4 232, viral load [VL] 37,600, on antiretroviral medication) and high blood pressure (controlled with atenolol). His doctor urged him to stop his weekend crack cocaine use and heavy drinking and referred him to addiction treatment. Bill was reluctant to go, hoping to cut down without outside help and to use only on days he was not visiting his son. After several primary care visits without significant change, he finally committed to going to outpatient treatment and Narcotics Anonymous (NA) meetings starting the following week. The following Friday was a payday, and he spent his entire check on crack cocaine. On Sunday, Bill was found dead in his single-room-occupancy hotel, having died of a myocardial infarction. A crack pipe and several beer bottles were on the table.[1]

Cerebrovascular System

In a study of adults ages 18–44 years discharged from Texas hospitals with stroke, cocaine abuse increased the risk of hemorrhagic or ischemic stroke, even after the study authors statistically controlled for other risk factors. METH increased the risk of hemorrhagic stroke and death (Westover et al. 2007).

Lungs

Smoking cocaine or METH exposes the lungs to the drug, contaminants, and fuel combustion products; long-term exposure can lead to pulmonary infiltrates, pulmonary edema, and severe asthma exacerbation (for review, see Tashkin 2001).

In a study of patients receiving treatment for tuberculosis (TB) in London (Story et al. 2008), crack users had higher odds of TB-positive smears than other illicit drug users (mostly heroin users), who in turn had higher odds of TB-positive smears than non–drug users. The study authors obtained these results after statistically controlling for other risk factors with multivariate analysis. This finding suggests that in addition to environmental conditions encountered by users of various illicit drugs (e.g., crowded, poorly ventilated shelters or jails), crack cocaine users' lung problems further increase their risk for TB (Story et al. 2008). Because of the high incidence of TB in stimulant- and other substance-using populations, residential drug treatment programs require TB screening before admission.

---

[1]This and other case examples in this chapter are a combination of several cases, with the name changed to protect confidentiality. This unfortunately all too common example illustrates how people can smoke crack for years, feel they can manage the medical and psychosocial consequences, and then suddenly have a fatal outcome.

Alonzo, a 50-year-old man with chronic obstructive pulmonary disease, was prescribed albuterol and a steroid inhaler (beclomethasone). He had stopped heavy drinking with the help of Alcoholics Anonymous 10 years earlier, but he smoked cigarettes (1 pack per day for the past 3 months, decreased from 3 packs per day for 32 years), marijuana (2 joints per day), and crack cocaine (several days a week). His nurse practitioner referred him to the health center's on-site mental health/substance abuse counselor, who provided motivational interviewing.

The counselor asked Alonzo how he felt about his lung disease. Alonzo said he was worried because his breathing had become so difficult that he could no longer walk to the main bus stop, and now had to wait for a local bus and then again for the downtown bus. When asked what he could do to improve his breathing, he said that at the end of last month he ran out of money and didn't smoke crack cocaine for a week. After this longer-than-usual break from crack cocaine, he noticed he was less winded and able to walk farther. During that week he still had cigarettes, which he purchased every few weeks in bulk, and got marijuana free from a friend. The counselor described how his lungs got a break from the toxins in the crack cocaine smoke. Alonzo acknowledged he needed to stop using crack cocaine (and was willing to give up the brief escape it gave him), would continue to cut down on cigarettes but was not ready to quit, and could not imagine giving up marijuana.

They then discussed treatment options. Because he was not ready to give up marijuana, he did not want to go to residential treatment. He decided to ask a friend to accompany him to NA meetings, and the counselor gave him information about two outpatient programs. In order not to smoke cigarettes after meetings or groups, Alonzo decided to stay inside the meeting room and speak with people there (rather than with the people who were smoking outside), then leave quickly. The counselor applauded him for committing to change two of the three substances that were harming his lungs.

Oral Health

Cocaine and particularly METH are associated with oral disease, including periodontal disease and tooth decay and loss. Stimulant use leads to vasoconstriction and dehydration (users often forget to drink water), which cause decreased salivary flow, resulting in increased gum disease and tooth decay. Poor dental hygiene and poor diet are also likely contributing factors (for review, see Hamamoto and Rhodus 2009).

Alonzo [see previous case example] said he was ready to quit crack cocaine now because he had finally made it to the dentist and had had several decayed teeth pulled. He stated that until he had dental work completed, he used crack cocaine in part for relief of tooth and gum pain.

Skin

Liu et al. (2010) provide a succinct review of skin problems resulting from use of cocaine, METH, and other drugs. Dehydration and nutritional deficiencies contribute to poor skin tone, skin dryness, and pruritis (itching); these occur with cocaine and METH, as well as with opioids, most of which can cause release of histamine. METH and cocaine users sometimes have hallucinations regarding their skin, including tactile hallucinations (*formication,* or a feeling of bugs under the skin) or visual hallucinations (e.g., seeing bugs or worms coming out of the skin) (Brewer et al. 2008). In response to itching or hallucinations, many users repeatedly scratch their skin, resulting in excoriations (open sores), infections, and scarring. Intravenous injection can cause track marks (hyperpigmented, linear scars along the injected veins), and subcutaneous injection ("skin popping") can result in deep, round scars (for review, see Liu et al. 2010). These marks and scars make it difficult to find veins for routine blood draws, and users often resort to injecting in more unsafe veins, such as in the neck. In addition, nonsterile injection is a major cause of infections of the skin (cellulitis) or other organs (see below).

> Alicia, a 37-year-old woman, was referred by Child Protective Services to outpatient treatment for METH dependence. She had recurrent major depression, had been introduced to METH by her husband at age 23, and started injecting it daily at age 28. METH helped her keep up with her two young children as a single parent. However, she felt ashamed because the track marks, sores, and dry skin made it obvious that she was an addict. When she was feeling depressed, she could not bear the looks she got from people at the pharmacy where she picked up new syringes, and so she just kept reusing her old syringes despite the scarring this caused.
>
> She came to her second session in tears because she said she could feel bugs crawling under her skin. She had told her doctor that wormlike things had started coming out of her skin, but her doctor did not provide any treatment or referrals. She begged her counselor to take her skin problems seriously and talk to her doctor. The counselor said that these problems would most likely go away when she stopped METH, and if not, she or the counselor could speak with her doctor then. She was able to stop crying, and discussed how she would ask her ex-husband (who had quit METH several years ago) to take the children for a week so that she could stop using and go through the crash associated with acute abstinence without worrying about her children.

Effects on Fetal Development

While findings related to the effect of stimulant use on birth defects have been mixed, several studies of prenatal stimulant exposure show neurological deficits even after statistically controlling for variables that might account for these deficits. In a study of newborns who were exposed antenatally to stimulants (cocaine, cocaine and an opiate, or METH) but had no other perinatal complications, 35% had brain abnormalities, a rate significantly more than the 5% rate of brain abnormalities observed among normally developing infants; these differences were not accounted for by other perinatal risk factors. The lesions in the drug-exposed group were focused in the basal ganglia, frontal lobes, and posterior fossa, probably related to the stimulants' vasoconstrictive effects (Dixon and Bejar 1989).

Controlled studies of long-term neurobehavioral deficits following prenatal cocaine exposure show mixed results. In a multisite longitudinal study of 1,227 infants (including 474 infants exposed to cocaine) at 1, 2, and 3 years of age, prenatal cocaine exposure was associated with motor, mental, and behavioral deficits, but the association disappeared after birth weight and environmental risks were controlled for (Messinger et al. 2004). In contrast, in a study of 880 nine-year-old children, the 277 children with prenatal cocaine exposure were more likely to be overweight and have high blood pressure, even after adjustment for demographics, maternal weight, other drug exposure, birth weight, diet, exercise, and television viewing habits (Shankaran et al. 2010).

Research on neurobehavioral deficits following prenatal METH exposure has begun more recently, with fewer studies and shorter follow-up periods. In a longitudinal study controlling for other variables, prenatal METH exposure was found to have dose-response relationships with neonatal neurobehavioral patterns of increased stress, decreased arousal, and poor quality of movement (Smith et al. 2008).

Children exposed to stimulants prenatally should receive regular developmental and mental health assessments and referrals as clinically indicated.

Injuries Resulting From Stimulant-Induced Behavior Changes

Stimulant use and resulting lack of sleep impair decision making and have been associated with increased risk taking while operating motor vehicles. However, associations with accidents and injuries are smaller than for alcohol or combined alcohol and drug use (see, e.g., Movig et al. 2004). Cocaine and METH do, however, increase risk of intentional violence toward others, including children, intimate partners, and friends. For example, in a retrospective study of clients in outpatient and residential drug abuse treatment programs, self-reported frequency of cocaine, stimulant, and heavy alcohol use were each associated with risk of violence toward and injury of an intimate partner, as well as violence and injury by an intimate partner, even after the study authors controlled for other risk factors, such as younger age and childhood physical abuse (Chermack et al. 2008). In contrast, these independent associations were not found for marijuana or for heroin or other opiates, none of which are as activating as alcohol and stimulants.

Effects of Cocaine and Methamphetamine on Infectious Disease Transmission

Infections Resulting From Adulterants

Many kinds of adulterants have been added to dilute or enhance the effects of cocaine or METH. Although many adulterants, such as caffeine or lactose, present a low risk of adverse events, some adulterants can be very toxic to humans. Levamisole, a livestock antiparasitic drug, has been added to bulk cocaine prior to shipment since 2002. Levamisole was detected in over 70% of illicit cocaine analyzed in the United States in July 2009 (Substance Abuse and Mental Health Services Administration 2009). Levamisole has been associated with agranulocytosis and neutropenia, resulting in dark skin sores that do not heal, and rapidly developing life-threatening infections. Cocaine users must be evaluated emergently if they develop infections (e.g., sore throat, mouth sores or thrush, or pneumonia in combination with fever, chills, weakness, or swollen glands), as these are conditions that can deteriorate rapidly (Substance Abuse and Mental Health Services Administration 2009) (for review and confirmed case, see Buchanan et al. 2010).

Infectious Disease Transmission Associated With Stimulant Injection

Many users inject cocaine or METH in order to get a large, immediate effect. Sharing injection equipment can transmit bacteria or viruses, including hepatitis C virus (HCV) and HIV—both serious chronic infections for which there is as yet no vaccine and no therapy that can eradicate the viruses. While HIV dies quickly outside the body, HCV can survive outside the body in dried blood for days. In addition, unsterile injection techniques or poor skin hygiene can result in skin and soft tissue infections (cellulitis), as well as infections of other organs, including the heart (endocarditis) or the brain (meningitis); the most common bacteria involved are *Staphylococcus aureus* (including methicillin-resistant *Staphylococcus aureus,* or MRSA) and streptococcal bacteria (for review, see Liu et al. 2010). Necrotizing fasciitis, an infection and destruction of the subcutaneous tissues, carries a high risk of sepsis and death.

Encouraging once-only syringe and needle use is the most effective way to reduce injection-related infectious disease in people who will not or cannot stop injecting drugs (Centers for Disease Control and Prevention 2005). Making syringes and needles available through syringe exchanges or pharmacies helps, but all injection drug users may not be reached through these channels. For example, in a study in San Francisco where there were numerous syringe exchanges, women who injected METH were more likely to report receptive syringe sharing and more than one syringe-sharing partner in the past 6 months, compared with women who injected other kinds of drugs, even after adjustment for other risk factors (Lorvick et al. 2006).

Infectious Diseases Related to Pipes or Straws

As with injection, many individuals smoke their cocaine (crack) or METH, as this produces a rapid and intense effect ("high"). In a study of 51 urban crack users, HCV RNA was found on one crack pipe (2%); its owner was HCV antibody positive and had a large sore on his lip (Fischer et al. 2008). This study showed that transmission from burns or sores (common on crack smokers' lips or hands) related to pipe smoking is possible. In another urban study, self-reported use of shared crack pipes with blood present correlated with having HCV in bivariate analyses, but not in multivariate analyses controlling for other risk factors such as age (Howe et al. 2005). In a study of injection drug users, crack cocaine smoking further increased their risk of acquiring HIV, after other variables were controlled for (DeBeck et al. 2009). In sum, although the pathways by which the reuse of previously used crack pipes or straws is associated with HCV and HIV have yet to be determined, it is safest to avoid used pipes and straws.

Infectious Diseases Transmitted by Stimulant-Related Sexual Risk Behaviors

Cocaine and METH use increase sexual risk behaviors that can transmit HIV and other sexually transmitted infections; HCV can also be transmitted sexually if there is contact with blood of an infected person. Numerous studies controlling for other risk factors have shown that cocaine and METH use are associated with unprotected sex, greater numbers of sex partners, and sexually transmitted infections, including HIV infection. Prolonged sex together with dehydration due to METH can result in dry skin and tears and cuts on the penis, anus, and vagina, increasing the risk of HIV and HCV transmission. In addition to sexual behavior, other variables may contribute, such as sexual networks with higher HIV prevalence and viral load due to difficulties with treatment access or adherence (for review, see Colfax et al. 2010).

Cocaine and METH users engage in high-risk sex for different reasons. Because the cocaine high is so brief, many quickly exhaust their financial resources and turn to other ways to get the drug, including exchanging sex for money or drugs, which may involve high numbers of partners, inconsistent condom use, and assault by partners (Sharpe 2005). In contrast, METH is often used in order to decrease inhibitions and prolong or enhance sex (Cheng et al. 2010).

> Ignacio, a 39-year-old man, had HIV/AIDS (CD4 210, VL 44), was receiving antiretroviral medication and consistently used condoms when having sex with his HIV-negative boyfriend of 4 years. Ignacio injected METH several times a week to improve his sexual functioning. One evening, when his boyfriend returned home, Ignacio was lying on the floor, complaining of back pain for the past several hours. He was also more suspicious than usual, asking the boyfriend repeatedly why he was out so late. He was taken to the emergency room, where he was diagnosed with meningitis caused by MRSA. After 2 weeks, Ignacio was transferred to the hospital's skilled nursing facility (SNF), where he stayed for nearly 2 months. While he was in the SNF, he committed to not using METH and attended on-site 12-step meetings. After discharge, he still had very little energy and had difficulty with sexual functioning with his boyfriend. After approximately 1 year of being abstinent from METH, Ignacio was eventually able to return to his previous level of activity.

Challenges in Medical Care of Stimulant Users With HIV

Although stimulant use can complicate the management of any medical condition, HIV is of most concern, both for individual stimulant users and for their communities. HIV increases incidence and severity of many other medical conditions, including cardiovascular disease and infectious diseases (for review, see Bruce and Altice 2007). Not receiving needed antiretroviral treatment increases transmission of HIV (Attia et al. 2009). As a result, any problems with access and adherence to HIV care not only affect stimulant users and their families but may contribute to the spread of HIV through entire populations.

Accelerated HIV Progression

METH has been shown to increase HIV replication in white blood cells in several in vitro studies (e.g., Toussi et al. 2009). Accelerated HIV progression has been shown in several studies of crack cocaine users. In a 30-month prospective study of 222 low-income drug users with HIV (Baum et al. 2009), crack cocaine users (50% of the sample) were more likely than other drug users to have their viral loads increase, and to have their CD4 cell count decline to less than 200 cells/mm^3 (qualifying for AIDS diagnosis), even after several other predictors (including alcohol use and receipt of antiretroviral medications) were controlled for by multivariate analysis. This finding was not accounted for by lower adherence among crack cocaine users, because it also occurred in the subgroup of users who were not receiving antiretroviral medications. Among patients who were taking HIV therapeutics, crack cocaine users were significantly less likely to achieve viral load control (e.g., 15% vs. 39% at 12-month follow-up). Although 54% of the sample drank alcohol (13% heavily), 35% of the sample used marijuana, and 14% used powder cocaine, none of these substances predicted HIV progression. The difference between crack and powder cocaine may have been in part because 35% of the crack cocaine users reported using daily or more often, compared with only 10% of the powder cocaine users. Because only 4% injected drugs, 6% used heroin, and less than 1% used METH, the study was not powered to evaluate the effect of these drugs. Thus, unfortunately, even though some active crack cocaine users are able to access health care and take their medications consistently, their HIV will progress more rapidly. This information may motivate some HIV-positive crack cocaine users to stop use of the drug.

Decreased Access to HIV Care

In a prospective study of adults with HIV accessing outreach programs in urban areas, cocaine use predicted ED visits, missed HIV medical appointments, and not being on antiretroviral medications despite CD4 counts of 350 cells/mm^3 or lower at 6-month follow-up (Sohler et al. 2007). These associations were similar to those found for injection drug use. Moreover, they were found even after adjustment for health status, insurance status, race, education, age, and gender. Those who had stopped using at 6-month follow-up did not differ significantly from nonusers in ED visits, missed medical appointments, or antiretroviral medication use. Other stimulants were used by only 14% of the sample and were unrelated to HIV care in this sample. In sum, although cocaine use disrupted HIV care, patients who stopped cocaine use were able to engage in regular health care.

Many cocaine users continue to use despite negative consequences and are not open to change. Although they may miss numerous appointments, it is still important to attempt to engage them in regular HIV care. Strategies include outreach, involvement of supportive family members, case management, and incentives for attendance. It is most helpful to provide multiple services in easily accessible locations, addressing the users' immediate priorities (e.g., food, housing assistance), along with needed medical services.

Interactions of HIV Medications With Cocaine and Methamphetamine

About 10% of cocaine is metabolized by the cytochrome P450 (CYP) family of liver enzymes, including CYP 3A4, which metabolizes numerous medications, including the non-nucleoside reverse transcriptase inhibitors and protease inhibitors used in most HIV medication regimens. Cocaine has been shown to induce CYP 3A4 metabolism in rodents (Pellinen et al. 1996). It is unknown whether and how much cocaine induces 3A4 metabolism in humans, and thus how much the doses may need to be increased.

Amphetamines and MDMA (3,4-methylenedioxymethamphetamine; ecstasy) are primarily metabolized by CYP 2D6, which the protease inhibitor ritonavir strongly inhibits. Given the case reports of near-fatal ecstasy overdoses after starting ritonavir (Henry and Hill 1998), it is important to encourage those with HIV disease to abstain from ecstasy use and, if they are unwilling to abstain, to remind them to check their reaction to a small amount first, because reactions to drugs differ between individuals and can change over time.

Many METH users take benzodiazepines to ease withdrawal. Ritonavir has been shown to inhibit CYP 3A4 metabolism of alprazolam (Xanax) (Greenblatt et al. 2000), and may also inhibit CYP 3A4 metabolism of clonazepam (Klonopin) and diazepam (Valium). Thus METH users who use benzodiazepines to "come down" should be warned they may become more sedated from the benzodiazepines than expected.

Many cocaine users are also opioid dependent and may be maintained on methadone or buprenorphine, the two opioid therapies that are U.S. Food and Drug Administration–approved for the treatment of opioid addiction. Chronic, regular cocaine use has been shown to be associated with reductions in plasma concentrations of buprenorphine (McCance-Katz et al. 2010a) and methadone (McCance-Katz and Mandell 2010). Methadone or buprenorphine in combination with cocaine use is not usually associated with opiate withdrawal. However, in patients who have other illnesses, such as HIV disease, that may require treatment with medications that also might induce metabolism of either methadone or buprenorphine, it is possible that opiate withdrawal might occur. Patients should receive treatment for cocaine use disorders when these disorders accompany opioid addiction and HIV disease. Opioid-maintained cocaine users should also be informed of the possibility of adverse drug interactions. When possible, use of medications that are less likely to be associated with adverse drug interactions (i.e., less likely to result in the induction of CYP 3A4) should be considered in opioid-maintained cocaine users (McCance-Katz et al. 2010b). METH has not been studied in combination with opioid pharmacotherapies to date.

Decreased Medication Adherence

Another difficulty with adherence to prescribed medications is that stimulant users tend to miss doses. They may report losing track of time, leaving home for days without taking their medication with them, or sleeping through their dose time. Cocaine and METH, as well as alcohol use, predict HAART (highly active antiretroviral therapy) nonadherence (for review, see Gruber et al. 2007). In a study of methadone maintenance patients (former or current heroin users), cocaine users had lower adherence to the HAART regimen than nonusers (27% vs. 68% of doses taken), and the proportion of patients in whom viral suppression was attained was lower (13% of users vs. 46% of nonusers) (Arnsten et al. 2002). Structure and supports can be helpful, such as the use of pill sorters, reminder systems, and directly administered therapy provided in locations patients get to frequently (e.g., housing programs, drop-in centers, methadone clinics).

> Mitch, a 39-year-old man with HIV/AIDS (CD4 290, VL 27,000), had smoked METH 3 days a week for 18 years. He developed a corneal ulcer and was referred to ophthalmology. However, he did not use the prescribed eyedrops consistently, stating that he often felt too tired. His corneal ulcer did not heal and developed permanent scarring, resulting in loss of vision in his left eye.

Cognitive Impairment

Among stimulant users with HIV, there are numerous causes of mild cognitive deficits (for review, see Anand et al. 2010). First, heavy cocaine and, especially, METH use can cause lasting mild cognitive impairments. Second, stimulant use increases the risk of head trauma and cerebrovascular accidents, which in turn lead to a wide range of cognitive impairments. Third, HIV crosses the blood-brain barrier within days of infection, eventually leading to HIV-associated neurocognitive disorders (HAND), such as HIV-associated dementia, mild neurocognitive impairment, and asymptomatic neurocognitive impairment. Cocaine and METH both increase HIV passage through the blood-brain barrier (Fiala et al. 2005; Mahajan et al. 2008). Finally, cognitive impairments can be caused by HIV-associated opportunistic infections (e.g., toxoplasmosis, cryptococcal meningitis), as well as by infections common among people with HIV as a result of shared risk factors (e.g., HCV, neurosyphilis). These cognitive impairments can contribute to difficulties with remembering and getting to appointments, taking medications as prescribed, and adopting safer sexual practices. When HIV-positive drug users show insight into the urgency of a needed action, but then do not follow through (e.g., regarding unsafe sex or drug use, missed appointments or medication doses), providers often have the impression it is because of low or mixed motivation, when actually it may be because of problems with executive functioning, impulsivity, or memory, or a combination of cognitive and motivational factors.

Behavioral and patient education interventions are more likely to be effective with these patients if information is presented multimodally (e.g., verbally as well as visually), reviewed frequently, provided in brief sessions (to reduce fatigue and distraction), and accompanied by real-world examples and at-home exercises, as well as checklists, reminders, mnemonics, and so forth. It is helpful to set up predictable periods of time when patients can drop in for services (e.g., Wednesday afternoons between 1:00 and 4:00 P.M.).

Stigma and Distrust

Because of the stigma and legal ramifications of illicit drug use, many drug users have had difficult interactions with the health care system, and expect to be treated in a punishing, withholding manner (Bruce and Altice 2007). As a result, many hide or underreport their drug use to health care providers. In response, many health care providers are suspicious and assume that patients are using far more than they say they are. Respecting drug users (in both words and actions) regardless of their readiness to stop using can help patients become more honest. If they come to a visit too intoxicated to participate, thank them for coming, discuss how they will get home safely, and talk about how they can get to the next visit without using on that day.

> Lisa, a 42-year-old woman, was brought by her sister to the emergency room. She had had a fever, headache, and stiff neck for 3 days. In the ED she had what appeared to be a seizure. She was admitted and diagnosed with cryptococcal meningitis and HIV. Her CD4 count was 10 (qualifying for a diagnosis of AIDS), and her viral load was 20,000, suggesting that she had had HIV for quite some time. Her admission urine toxicology screen was positive for cocaine metabolite, and she eventually admitted to smoking crack cocaine several days a week since age 17.
>
> After a month she was discharged to the outpatient clinic's HIV treatment engagement program. At her first visit, she had used crack cocaine but made it in to the appointment because her sister brought her. She could not sit still, stood up and paced around, and said she had a lot of things to do and needed to go. The nurse thanked her and her sister for coming and scheduled the next visit for several days later. Lisa agreed to not smoke crack cocaine before her clinic appointments.

At the next visit, the nurse continued the HIV education and explained to Lisa how her health would improve if she started antiretroviral medication and stopped crack cocaine use. She understood that she had HIV disease, but she said that she was feeling better, so it did not make sense to her to take medication. After three visits, one of them with her sister present, she agreed to take antiretroviral medication. Her primary care doctor met with Lisa and selected a medication regimen with her.

Lisa then met weekly with the nurse, who reviewed the past week's adherence, problem-solved how to prevent missed doses, and gave her a pill organizer containing each day's medications for the next week, along with several emergency doses in case she did not come in on the scheduled day. If Lisa came to the clinic on the scheduled day, she received a grocery or thrift store gift card. At each visit she also met with a social worker, who helped her apply for Social Security disability and started motivational interviewing regarding Lisa's crack cocaine use.

KEY CLINICAL CONCEPTS

- Although extreme examples of health problems from cocaine or methamphetamine (METH) use are often not credible to users, many well-controlled studies now link stimulant use to various medical problems, some of them fatal. Knowledge of these problems can help stimulant users and health care providers respond to symptoms earlier.

- Stimulant overdose manifests initially with symptoms such as agitation, increased heart rate, and hyperthermia, which can eventually lead to rhabdomyolysis and renal failure.

- Long-term stimulant use increases the risk of hypertension, atherosclerosis, vasospasm, thrombosis formation, myocardial infarction, and stroke. Rarely, vasoconstriction can also cause corneal ulcers and scarring, resulting in blindness.

- Smoking crack or METH harms the lungs, exacerbates asthma and chronic obstructive pulmonary disease, and increases vulnerability to tuberculosis.

- Cocaine and, especially, METH can cause gum disease and tooth decay via vasoconstriction, dehydration, reduced salivary flow, poor dental hygiene, and poor diet.

- Cocaine and METH use can lead to dehydration and nutritional deficiencies that result in dry, itchy skin. In addition, some users have tactile or visual hallucinations involving their skin (e.g., feeling bugs under their skin).

- Children exposed prenatally to cocaine or METH are at increased risk for neurobehavioral problems and should receive regular developmental and mental health assessments and referrals as needed.

- Cocaine and METH use are associated with increased risk of violence toward and from intimate partners.

- Unprotected sex, used needles/syringes, and possibly pipes can transmit HIV and hepatitis C virus. Poor skin hygiene when injecting can result in infections of the skin (abscesses), heart (endocarditis), or other organs. The adulterant levamisole, found in most cocaine, can result in neutropenia and life-threatening infections.

- Cocaine and possibly METH increase HIV disease progression, and thus it is important to engage stimulant users in both HIV care and addiction treatment as early as possible.

Resources

Bruce RD, Altice FL: Clinical care of the HIV-infected drug user. Infect Dis Clin North Am 21:149–179, 2007.
Detailed medical description of identification and treatment of infectious diseases common in drug users, including HIV. Review of methadone and buprenorphine treatment for opioid dependence and their interactions with HIV medications.

Bungay V, Johnson JL, Varcoe C, et al: Women's health and use of crack cocaine in context: structural and "everyday" violence. Int J Drug Policy 21:321–329, 2010

Waller JM, Feramisco JD, Alberta-Wszolek L, et al: Cocaine-associated retiform purpura and neutropenia: is levamisole the culprit? J Am Acad Dermatol 63:530–535, 2010.
Helpful cases and color pictures of lesions related to possible life-threatening consequences of levamisole in cocaine.

http://www.dancesafe.org/health-and-safety/heatstroke.
User-friendly instructions for prevention and first aid for heatstroke.

http://www.kci.org.
Methamphetamine information for users, family members, affected communities. Includes links to PowerPoint presentations at scientific meetings.

http://www.erowid.org.
Information about various psychoactive drugs, medical effects, user experiences, and drug testing.

http://www.projectinform.org.
The health information section has easy-to-read PDFs on various HIV health topics and medications, including a link to tables on HIV medication interactions with street drugs.

References

Anand P, Springer SA, Copenhaver MM, et al: Neurocognitive impairment and HIV risk factors: a reciprocal relationship. AIDS Behav 14:1213–1226, 2010

Arnsten JH, Demas PA, Grant RW, et al: Impact of active drug use on antiretroviral therapy adherence and viral suppression in HIV-infected drug users. J Gen Intern Med 17:377–381, 2002

Attia S, Egger M, Muller M, et al: Sexual transmission of HIV according to viral load and antiretroviral therapy: systematic review and meta-analysis. AIDS 23:1397–1404, 2009

Baum MK, Rafie C, Lai S, et al: Crack-cocaine use accelerates HIV disease progression in a cohort of HIV-positive drug users. J Acquir Immune Defic Syndr 50:93–99, 2009

Brewer JD, Meves A, Bostwick J, et al: Cocaine abuse: dermatologic manifestations and therapeutic approaches. J Am Acad Dermatol 59:483–487, 2008

Bruce RD, Altice FL: Clinical care of the HIV-infected drug user. Infect Dis Clin North Am 21:149–179, 2007

Buchanan JA, Oyer RJ, Patel NR, et al: A confirmed case of agranulocytosis after use of cocaine contaminated with levamisole. J Med Toxicol 6:160–164, 2010

Centers for Disease Control and Prevention: Access to sterile syringes. December 2005. Available at: http://www.cdc.gov/idu/facts/aed_idu_acc.htm. Accessed March 22, 2011.

Cheng WS, Garfein RS, Semple SJ, et al: Binge use and sex and drug behaviors among HIV(–), heterosexual methamphetamine users in San Diego. Subst Use Misuse 45:116–133, 2010

Chermack ST, Murray RL, Walton MA, et al: Partner aggression among men and women in substance use disorder treatment: correlates of psychological and physical aggression and injury. Drug Alcohol Depend 98:35–44, 2008

Colfax G, Santos GM, Chu P, et al: Amphetamine-group substances and HIV. Lancet 736:458–474, 2010

Darke S, Kaye S, McKetin R, et al: Major physical and psychological harms of methamphetamine use. Drug Alcohol Rev 27:253–262, 2008

DeBeck K, Kerr T, Li K, et al: Smoking of crack cocaine as a risk factor for HIV infection among people who use injection drugs. CMAJ 181:585–589, 2009

Diercks DB, Fonarow GC, Kirk JD, et al: Illicit stimulant use in a United States heart failure population presenting to the emergency department (from the Acute Decompensated Heart Failure National Registry Emergency Module). Am J Cardiol 102:1216–1219, 2008

Dixon SD, Bejar R: Echoencephalographic findings in neonates associated with maternal cocaine and methamphetamine use: incidence and clinical correlates. J Pediatr 115:770–778, 1989

Fiala M, Eshleman AJ, Cashman J, et al: Cocaine increases human immunodeficiency virus type 1 neuroinvasion through remodeling brain microvascular endothelial cells. J Neurovirol 11:281–291, 2005

Fischer B, Powis J, Firestone CM, et al: Hepatitis C virus transmission among oral crack users: viral detection on crack paraphernalia. Eur J Gastroenterol Hepatol 20:29–32, 2008

Graham JK, Hanzlick R: Accidental drug deaths in Fulton County, Georgia, 2002: characteristics, case management and certification issues. Am J Forensic Med Pathol 29:224–230, 2008

Greenblatt DJ, von Moltke LL, Harmatz JS, et al: Alprazolam-ritonavir interaction: implications for product labeling. Clin Pharmacol Ther 67:335–341, 2000

Gruber VA, Sorensen JL, Haug NA: Psychosocial predictors of adherence to highly active antiretroviral therapy: practical implications. J HIV AIDS Soc Serv 6:23–37, 2007

Hamamoto DT, Rhodus NL: Methamphetamine abuse and dentistry. Oral Dis 15:27–37, 2009

Hazin R, Cadet JL, Kahook MY, et al: Ocular manifestations of crystal methamphetamine use. Neurotox Res 15:187–191, 2009

Henry JA, Hill IR: Fatal interaction between ritonavir and MDMA. Lancet 352:1751–1752, 1998

Howe CJ, Fuller CM, Ompad DC, et al: Association of sex, hygiene and drug equipment sharing with hepatitis C virus infection among non-injecting drug users in New York City. Drug Alcohol Depend 79:389–395, 2005

Kaye S, McKetin R, Duflou J, et al: Methamphetamine and cardiovascular pathology: a review of the evidence. Addiction 102:1204–1211, 2007

Kaye S, Darke S, Duflou J, et al: Methamphetamine-related fatalities in Australia: demographics, circumstances, toxicology and major organ pathology. Addiction 103:1353–1360, 2008

Lai S, Fishman EK, Lai H, et al: Long-term cocaine use and antiretroviral therapy are associated with silent coronary artery disease in African Americans with HIV infection who have no cardiovascular symptoms. Clin Infect Dis 46:600–610, 2008

Lan KC, Lin YF, Yu FC, et al: Clinical manifestations and prognostic features of acute methamphetamine intoxication. J Formos Med Assoc 97:528–533, 1998

Liu SW, Lien MH, Fenske NA: The effects of alcohol and drug abuse on the skin. Clin Dermatol 28:391–399, 2010

Lorvick J, Martinez A, Gee L, et al: Sexual and injection risk among women who inject methamphetamine in San Francisco. J Urban Health 83:497–505, 2006

Mahajan SD, Aalinkeel R, Sykes DE, et al: Methamphetamine alters blood brain barrier permeability via modulation of tight junction expression: implication for HIV-1 neuropathogenesis in the context of drug abuse. Brain Res 1203:133–148, 2008

McCance-Katz EF, Mandell TW: Drug interactions of clinical importance with methadone and buprenorphine. Am J Addict 19:2–3, 2010

McCance-Katz EF, Rainey PM, Moody DE: Effect of cocaine use on buprenorphine pharmacokinetics in humans. Am J Addict 19:38–46, 2010a

McCance-Katz EF, Sullivan LE, Nallani S: Drug interactions of clinical importance between the opioids, methadone and buprenorphine, and frequently prescribed medications: a review. Am J Addict 19:4–16, 2010b

McGuinness TM, Pollack D: Parental methamphetamine abuse and children. J Pediatr Health Care 22:152–158, 2008

Messinger DS, Bauer CR, Das A, et al: The maternal lifestyle study: cognitive, motor and behavioral outcomes of cocaine-exposed and opiate-exposed infants through three years of age. Pediatrics 113:1677–1685, 2004

Moliterno DJ, Willard JE, Lange RA, et al: Coronary artery vasoconstriction induced by cocaine, cigarette smoking or both. N Engl J Med 330:454–459, 1994

Movig KL, Mathijssen MP, Nagel PH, et al: Psychoactive substance use and the risk of motor vehicle accidents. Accid Anal Prev 36:631–636, 2004

Pellinen P, Stenbäck F, Kojo A, et al: Regenerative changes in hepatic morphology and enhanced expression of CYP2B10 and CYP3A during daily administration of cocaine. Hepatology 23:515–523, 1996

Phillips K, Luk A, Soor GS, et al: Cocaine cardiotoxicity: a review of the pathophysiology, pathology and treatment options. Am J Cardiovasc Drugs 9:177–196, 2009

Richards JR, Johnson EB, Stark RW, et al: Methamphetamine abuse and rhabdomyolysis in the ED: a 5-year-study. Am J Emerg Med 17:681–685, 1999

Ruttenber AJ, McAnally HB, Wetli CV: Cocaine-associated rhabdomyolysis and excited delirium: different stages of the same syndrome. Am J Forensic Med Pathol 20:120–127, 1999

Shankaran S, Bann CM, Bauer CR, et al: Prenatal cocaine exposure and BMI and blood pressure at 9 years of age. J Hypertens 28:1166–1175, 2010

Sharpe TT: Behind the Eight-Ball: Sex for Crack Cocaine Exchange and Poor Black Women. New York, Taylor & Francis, 2005

Smith LM, Lagasse LL, Derauf C, et al: Prenatal methamphetamine use and neonatal neurobehavioral outcome. Neurotoxicol Teratol 30:20–28, 2008

Sohler NL, Wong MD, Cunningham WE, et al: Type and pattern of illicit drug use and access to health care services for HIV-infected people. AIDS Patient Care STDS 21 (suppl 1):S68–S76, 2007

Story A, Bothamley G, Hayward A: Crack cocaine and infectious tuberculosis. Emerg Infect Dis 14:1466–1469, 2008

Substance Abuse and Mental Health Services Administration: Nationwide public health alert issued concerning life-threatening risk posed by cocaine laced with veterinary anti-parasite drug. News release, September 1, 2009. Available at: http://www.samhsa.gov/newsroom/advisories/090921vet5101.aspx. Accessed March 23, 2011.

Tashkin DP: Airway effects of marijuana, cocaine, and other inhaled illicit agents. Curr Opin Pulm Med 7:43–61, 2001

Toussi SS, Joseph A, Zheng JA, et al: Short communication: methamphetamine treatment increases in vitro and in vivo HIV replication. AIDS Res Hum Retroviruses 254:1117–1121, 2009

Westover AN, McGride S, Haley RW: Stroke in young adults who abuse amphetamines or cocaine: a population-based study of hospitalized patients. Arch Gen Psychiatry 64:495–502, 2007

Chapter 8

Summary and Future Directions

Thomas F. Newton, M.D.
Colin N. Haile, M.D., Ph.D.

This volume presents clear evidence that significant progress is being made toward developing treatments for stimulant dependence. Stimulant dependence is increasingly considered a brain disease, and this view has refocused attention on empirically validated medication treatments combined with behavior therapy. Neuroimaging studies consistently identify stable functional changes in stimulant-dependent individuals, suggesting that vulnerability to stimulant dependence may be a preexisting or acquired trait. Recent insight into these neurochemical deficiencies guides current approaches to combating this pernicious disease. Identifying medication treatments to correct the neurochemical abnormalities underlying stimulant dependence is an approach shared with other fields of mainstream medicine.

Constant vigilance regarding changes in epidemiology, fluctuations in drug availability, and changes in drug trafficking patterns is essential to understanding emerging new drug abuse patterns. Cocaine and methamphetamine (METH) and amphetamine (AMPH) differ greatly, so shifts in the predominant drug of abuse can have important consequences. The drugs have different effects on neurotransmitters and greatly differ in their pharmacokinetic characteristics. It is these differences that explain their characteristic reinforcing effects and addictive liabilities and that help inform research on the types of medications likely to be effective. Similar to current trends in the management of depression, in which psychotherapy is combined with medication treatment, recent advances in and validation of behavioral interventions like contingency management, cognitive-behavioral therapy (CBT), and motivational interviewing will undoubtedly improve treatment of stimulant dependence.

The criminal justice system's shift away from punitive action and toward more humane treatment, including medical management and treatment for stimulant dependence, has many far-reaching benefits. For example, major depression and psychosis are common in cocaine- and METH/AMPH-dependent individuals, and may continue after drug use has stopped. These disorders require proper psychiatric care that is often unavailable in prisons.

Mechanisms of Action and Subjective and Physiological Effects

Cocaine and METH/AMPH have different mechanisms of action and subjective and physiological effects (Newton et al. 2005). Cocaine produces relatively brief increases in synaptic levels of dopamine (DA), norepinephrine (NE), and serotonin by blocking reuptake, whereas METH and AMPH produce prolonged increases in the levels of these neurotransmitters by inducing release. Secondary effects of both include disruption of central glutamate (GLU) homeostasis, which may play a role in drug relapse. Neurotransmitter changes within the mesocorticolimbic system correlate with psychostimulant euphoric effects and drug craving. Cocaine and METH/AMPH adversely affect cellular mechanisms involved in neural plasticity, and this effect is linked to long-lasting changes in learning and memory. These memory impairments may contribute to relapse in humans. Chronic use produces maladaptive changes in brain structure and function. Neuroimaging studies show that cocaine-dependent individuals have decreased DA synthesis, low endogenous DA levels, reduced DA release, and reduced D_2/D_3 receptor availability. In contrast, striatal dopamine transporter (DAT) number and function are *increased,* and this contributes to reductions in postsynaptic DA binding because of rapid reuptake. Counter to what might be expected, cocaine-dependent individuals have blunted subjective "high" responses to stimulants and decreased striatal activation, yet increased sensitivity to memory cues associated with drug taking (Volkow et al. 2010). Alcohol-dependent individuals also display blunted subjective responses to drugs that target receptors implicated in alcohol's effects, and are also hypersensitive to cues associated with alcohol consumption (Volkow et al. 1993).

These data suggest that selective brain receptors and circuits that control drug responsivity are usurped in drug-dependent individuals, and this may be common across drug classes. Indeed, METH/AMPH dependence is associated with decreased striatal DAT and vesicular monoamine transporter–2 expression. Studies indicate that METH/AMPH-induced neurotoxicity is partly caused by DA-mediated oxidative stress, excitotoxicity, hyperthermia, and neuroinflammation. Logically, anti-inflammatory agents and medications that enhance cortical activation and cognition have shown promise for METH/AMPH dependence. Taken together, these findings suggest that different combinations of medications that correct neurotransmitter tone and/or counter neurotoxicity may be needed to ameliorate the many deficits associated with cocaine or METH/AMPH.

Recently available research tools to probe previously neglected neurotransmitter systems have revealed new insights into the effects of stimulants on the brain and refocused the direction of research. Studies show a greater role for NEergic and GLUergic mechanisms in stimulant dependence than previously thought. Older medications that may have central effects on NE and GLU have been assessed for stimulant dependence; these agents already have indications for other diseases, potentially decreasing the time needed before they may be used clinically. For example, the antibiotic minocycline increases central GLU levels and blocks METH's deleterious effects on the DAT (Hashimoto et al. 2007), attenuates AMPH's subjective effects in humans (Sofuoglu et al. 2011), and has been used successfully to treat METH dependence with psychosis (Tanibuchi et al. 2010). Similarly, the antibiotic ceftriaxone (which alters GLU levels) has been shown to block relapse to cocaine self-administration in animal models (Knackstedt et al. 2010), and N-acetylcysteine, a medication used to treat acetaminophen overdose, also normalizes GLU levels and decreases cocaine craving in humans (LaRowe et al. 2006; Mardikian et al. 2007). Disulfiram was originally indicated to treat alcohol dependence but has been found to significantly reduce cocaine use in humans. Naltrexone, a medication that targets the opioid system and is indicated in the treatment of alcohol and opioid dependence, significantly attenuates the subjective effects of AMPH and reduces craving and AMPH use in humans (Jayaram-Lindström et al. 2004, 2008). Studies continue to support the wake-promoting medication modafinil, which affects DA and NE levels but also significantly increases GLU neurotransmission, for stimulant dependence (De La Garza et al. 2010).

Taken together, these research findings have led to a greater understanding of the effects of stimulants on the human brain, which has enabled hypothesis-driven reassessment of medications with other indications as possible treatments for stimulant dependence.

Polydrug Abuse

Most stimulant-dependent individuals use other drugs of abuse, including nicotine. These drug combinations also increase the incidence of adverse events. Successful treatment of polydrug users continues to be a challenge. For instance, a large proportion of stimulant-dependent individuals are also nicotine dependent, and this may alter therapeutic response to some treatments. All drugs of abuse share common neurobiological substrates; thus, medications for smoking cessation are being tested for cocaine dependence. Medications that have shown promise as treatments for dependence on stimulants, such as modafinil and topiramate, unfortunately enhance nicotine's subjective effects. It is unknown whether modafinil or topiramate increases or decreases smoking in stimulant-dependent individuals. Similarly, cannabis, generally considered to be a depressant, enhances cocaine's stimulant subjective and physiological effects, and alcohol enhances cocaine and METH's effects. These drug combinations, compared with a single drug of abuse, have synergistic adverse effects on brain morphology, neurocognition, and general overall health that result in continued relapse and chronic debility. Addressing multiple systems–level pathology may require multiple medications combined with behavior therapy.

Effects on Overall Health and Well-Being

Cocaine and METH/AMPH dependence adversely affect overall health and well-being on many levels. For example, stimulant overdose may lead to renal failure, which requires lifelong dialysis. Hypertension, myocardial infarction, and stroke are common in the stimulant-dependent population. Gum disease and tooth decay associated with METH use are linked to cardiovascular heart disease. Smoking is the preferred route of administration for cocaine and METH, and smoking is linked to lung disease and increased risk of tuberculosis. Viruses such as HIV and hepatitis C are transmitted through risky sexual behavior and sharing of syringes for intravenous injection and pipes used to smoke crack cocaine or METH. Cocaine and METH use also compromise immune function, allowing diseases to progress and hastening morbidity and mortality. A wide variety of adulterant agents are found in cocaine and METH/AMPH, and some are known to cause immunosuppression and death (e.g., levamisole). Primary care providers for the most part deliver medical care to this population and are constantly challenged by the pathophysiology associated with chronic cocaine and METH/AMPH use and dependence. Programs are needed to educate caregivers about adverse effects of stimulant addiction on general overall health measures. Such efforts may facilitate proper diagnosis and treatment and avert chronic and progressive morbidity.

Future Directions

Although presently no pharmacotherapies are indicated for the treatment of stimulant dependence, the evidence presented in this volume suggests that efficacious treatments for stimulant addiction may soon be forthcoming. However, a number of questions still remain to be answered, and certain policies proven not to work need to be reconsidered. Although much improved, present drug policies point toward a need for more harm reduction–oriented public policies in dealing with drug dependence in general and stimulant dependence in particular. This is especially true as addiction is increasingly conceptualized as a chronic disease. Implied within the chronic disease model is the recognition that relapses will be common, and this necessitates increased emphasis on harm reduction rather than administrative remedies (i.e., law enforcement). Harm reduction approaches advocate decreased rates of incarceration and emphasize the need for medical management. This approach may lead to decreased health care costs in general by preventing secondary medical conditions and psychiatric illness comorbidity. European drug substitution programs for opioid dependence show beneficial effects on overall health, decreased disease transmission, reduction in crime, and reduced overall mortality and morbidity associated with drug use (Michels et al. 2007; Nordt and Stohler 2006, 2010). Likewise, recently published studies evaluating U.S. programs for cocaine dependence that use harm reduction techniques show similar positive effects, including significant reduction in drug use, fewer sex partners, and reduced crime (e.g., Bowser et al. 2010). Countries that have a sizeable population of intravenous drug users are addressing the adverse consequences of this route of administration, such as increased disease transmission (Kerr et al. 2010; Mravík et al. 2011). More extensive and long-term unbiased studies assessing the efficacy of harm reduction techniques for stimulant dependence are needed.

Future addiction medicine treatments should take a more individualized approach based on 1) drug dependence subtype, 2) gender, 3) race, 4) medical and psychiatric comorbidities, 5) functional brain deficiencies (i.e., DA, NE tone, or memory deficits), and 6) pharmacogenetic profile. For example, drug-dependent individuals who binge may require different therapies than do chronic maintenance users. Much evidence supports the notion that drug use, responses to stimulants, and development of comorbidities significantly differ between males and females (Cotto et al. 2010; Dluzen and Liu 2008; Mahoney et al. 2010). Similar to gender effects, race is also associated with whether an individual prefers cocaine or METH/AMPH. This difference in stimulant choice is not dependent on geography, cost, or drug availability but does appear to be mediated by genetically based differences in the affinity of striatal DAT for the drug (Bousman et al. 2010; Fowler et al. 2008). Psychosis associated with METH/AMPH use is more prevalent in Asian populations compared with other populations and eventually becomes chronic in a substantial minority of those affected. The long-term prognosis of METH/AMPH-dependent individuals who experience psychosis when drug use is stopped is not promising; however, some standard psychiatric therapies have shown some treatment efficacy (Grelotti et al. 2010; Kittirattanapaiboon et al. 2010).

As previous chapters have extensively detailed, cocaine and METH/AMPH-dependent individuals have fairly consistent functional brain deficiencies, generally related to learning and memory, that may involve decreased DA tone. Logically, cognitive enhancers and other medications that increase working memory have been shown to either reduce the subjective effects of stimulants or decrease use in outpatient studies (Anderson et al. 2009; Herin et al. 2010; Kalechstein et al. 2010; Sofuoglu 2010). Advances in pharmacology and genetics research continue to transform the way medications are used in clinical practice. Pharmacokinetic and pharmacodynamic variability are heavily influenced by genetic background, and thus, the goal of pharmacogenetics is to correlate drug response with an individual's genetic makeup. Attention to genetic background can improve treatment outcome for other psychiatric diseases (Zhang and Malhotra 2011). Recent research relating single-nucleotide polymorphisms (SNPs) and drug responses also supports using a pharmacogenetic approach to improve pharmacotherapeutic efficacy for stimulant dependence (Haile and Kosten 2009; Haile et al. 2007, 2009). Greater understanding is still needed, however, before we can develop individualized treatments based on SNPs or other gene variants that may alter the pharmacokinetic or pharmacodynamic action of a given medication.

Future developments may allow use of pharmacotherapeutics aimed at blocking or reversing synaptic plasticity associated with stimulant dependence. Only very recently have we identified the possibility that medications to treat inflammation and toxicity resulting from stimulant abuse and dependence may prove effective therapies for reducing use (Hashimoto et al. 2004; LaRowe et al. 2006; Sekine et al. 2008). Similarly, medications with neurotrophic actions or those that induce neurotrophic factor release may reverse drug-induced changes, enhance cognitive functioning, and reduce oxidative stress (Bradley et al. 2010; Krasnova and Cadet 2009). Thus, it is likely that more than one medication will be needed to address whichever particular facet of stimulant dependence predominates.

Novel therapeutic targets, technology, and strategies are needed to better address the lack of progress in treating stimulant dependence. Fortunately, new treatment modalities have been developed in the last decade, such as vaccines to target stimulant drugs, preventing access to the central nervous system and offering a greater advantage for sustained abstinence (Kinsey et al. 2010; Martell et al. 2009). With future development, enhancing enzymes that facilitate the quick inactivation of cocaine in the periphery may also be useful (Gao et al. 2010; Lockridge et al. 2005). These peripheral therapies may prove advantageous to augment pharmacological interventions. Technological advances in utilizing virtual environments meant to desensitize cue-induced drug craving, coupled with contingency management or CBT, have shown recent promise as adjunct nonpharmacological therapies for stimulant dependence (Culbertson et al. 2010; Vocci and Montoya 2009). Critical focus on the development of better preclinical models that demonstrate some predictive validity regarding possible medications for stimulant dependence has recently helped clarify medication development objectives (Yahyavi-Firouz-Abadi and See 2009). Assessing older drugs that have indications for other diseases, yet act on neurobiological substrates that mediate stimulant withdrawal, craving, and rewarding effects, continues to be an effective strategy for medication development for stimulant dependence (De La Garza et al. 2008; Newton et al. 2010). Research on a variety of fronts is moving us closer to identifying effective treatments for stimulant dependence, and improved understanding of the genetic and biological substrates on which these treatments act will facilitate their development.

KEY CLINICAL CONCEPTS

- Our understanding of stimulant dependence in general, and of the way these drugs exert their neurobiological effects in particular, has progressed rapidly over the last decade, mainly because of advances in technology such as neuroimaging.

- Cocaine and methamphetamine/amphetamine (METH/AMPH) differ in their pharmacokinetic and pharmacodynamic profiles, which relate directly to their use, associated comorbidities, and effects on overall health.

- Numerous older drugs that have an indication for other diseases have been reassessed as treatments for stimulant dependence, with some showing promise.

- Harm reduction strategies advocate increasing treatment opportunities, rather than emphasizing incarceration. The present drug law policies have failed to curb illicit drug consumption. Harm reduction techniques may decrease disease transmission, reduce crime, decrease overall mortality and morbidity, and result in reduced health care costs associated with drug use.

- Recent research on novel therapeutic approaches acting outside of the central nervous system includes studies of vaccines against drugs of abuse (including cocaine and METH/AMPH) and investigations into enzymes that speed the elimination of these drugs from the body.

- Future treatment of stimulant dependence using an individualized pharmacogenetic approach may increase medication efficacy and reduce adverse drug events.

Resources

National Institute on Drug Abuse treatment options overview
http://www .nida.nih.gov/infofacts/treatmeth.html

Medication development
http://irp.drugabuse.gov/branches.html

Substance abuse treatment facility locator map
http://dasis3.samhsa.gov/

College on Problems of Drug Dependence
http://www.cpdd.vcu.edu/index.html

Society for Neuroscience
http://www.sfn.org/

References

Anderson AL, Reid MS, Li SH, et al: Modafinil for the treatment of cocaine dependence. Drug Alcohol Depend 104:133–139, 2009

Bousman CA, Glatt SJ, Cherner M, et al: Preliminary evidence of ethnic divergence in associations of putative genetic variants for methamphetamine dependence. Psychiatry Res 178:295–298, 2010

Bowser BP, Jenkins-Barnes T, Dillard-Smith C, et al: Harm reduction for drug abusing ex-offenders: outcome of the California prevention and education project MORE project. J Evid Based Soc Work 7:15–29, 2010

Bradley LH, Fuqua J, Richardson A, et al: Dopamine neuron stimulating actions of a GDNF propeptide. PloS One 5:e9752, 2010

Cotto JH, Davis E, Dowling GJ, et al: Gender effects on drug use, abuse, and dependence: a special analysis of results from the National Survey on Drug Use and Health. Gend Med 7:402–413, 2010

Culbertson C, Nicolas S, Zaharovits I, et al: Methamphetamine craving induced in an online virtual reality environment. Pharmacol Biochem Behav 96:454–460, 2010

De La Garza R [2nd], Shoptaw S, Newton TF: Evaluation of the cardiovascular and subjective effects of rivastigmine in combination with methamphetamine in methamphetamine-dependent human volunteers. Int J Neuropsychopharmacol 11:729–741, 2008

De La Garza R 2nd, Zorick T, London ED, et al: Evaluation of modafinil effects on cardiovascular, subjective, and reinforcing effects of methamphetamine in methamphetamine-dependent volunteers. Drug Alcohol Depend 106:173–180, 2010

Dluzen DE, Liu B: Gender differences in methamphetamine use and responses: a review. Gend Med 5:24–35, 2008

Fowler JS, Volkow ND, Logan J, et al: Fast uptake and long-lasting binding of methamphetamine in the human brain: comparison with cocaine. Neuroimage 43:756–763, 2008

Gao Y, Orson FM, Kinsey B, et al: The concept of pharmacologic cocaine interception as a treatment for drug abuse. Chem Biol Interact 187:421–424, 2010

Grelotti DJ, Kanayama G, Pope HG Jr: Remission of persistent methamphetamine-induced psychosis after electroconvulsive therapy: presentation of a case and review of the literature. Am J Psychiatry 167:17–23, 2010

Haile CN, Kosten TR: The potential of pharmacogenomics to treat drug addiction. Pharmacogenomics 10:1883–1886, 2009

Haile CN, Kosten TR, Kosten TA: Genetics of dopamine and its contribution to cocaine addiction. Behav Genet 37:119–145, 2007

Haile CN, Kosten TR, Kosten TA: Pharmacogenetic treatments for drug addiction: cocaine, amphetamine and methamphetamine. Am J Drug Alcohol Abuse 35:161–177, 2009

Hashimoto K, Tsukada H, Nishiyama S, et al: Protective effects of N-acetyl-L-cysteine on the reduction of dopamine transporters in the striatum of monkeys treated with methamphetamine. Neuropsychopharmacology 29:2018–2023, 2004

Hashimoto K, Tsukada H, Nishiyama S, et al: Protective effects of minocycline on the reduction of dopamine transporters in the striatum after administration of methamphetamine: a positron emission tomography study in conscious monkeys. Biol Psychiatry 61:577–581, 2007

Herin DV, Rush CR, Grabowski J: Agonist-like pharmacotherapy for stimulant dependence: preclinical, human laboratory, and clinical studies. Ann N Y Acad Sci 1187:76–100, 2010

Jayaram-Lindström N, Wennberg P, Hurd YL, et al: Effects of naltrexone on the subjective response to amphetamine in healthy volunteers. J Clin Psychopharmacol 24:665–669, 2004

Jayaram-Lindström N, Konstenius M, Eksborg S, et al: Naltrexone attenuates the subjective effects of amphetamine in patients with amphetamine dependence. Neuropsychopharmacology 33:1856–1863, 2008

Kalechstein AD, De La Garza R 2nd, Newton TF: Modafinil administration improves working memory in methamphetamine-dependent individuals who demonstrate baseline impairment. Am J Addict 19:340–344, 2010

Kerr T, Hayashi K, Fairbairn N, et al: Expanding the reach of harm reduction in Thailand: experiences with a drug user-run drop-in centre. Int J Drug Policy 21:255–258, 2010

Kinsey BM, Kosten TR, Orson FM: Anti-cocaine vaccine development. Expert Rev Vaccines 9:1109–1114, 2010

Kittirattanapaiboon P, Mahatnirunkul S, Booncharoen H, et al: Long-term outcomes in methamphetamine psychosis patients after first hospitalisation. Drug Alcohol Rev 29:456–461, 2010

Knackstedt LA, Melendez RI, Kalivas PW: Ceftriaxone restores glutamate homeostasis and prevents relapse to cocaine seeking. Biol Psychiatry 67:81–84, 2010

Krasnova IN, Cadet JL: Methamphetamine toxicity and messengers of death. Brain Res Rev 60:379–407, 2009

LaRowe SD, Mardikian P, Malcolm R, et al: Safety and tolerability of N-acetylcysteine in cocaine-dependent individuals. Am J Addict 15:105–110, 2006

Lockridge O, Schopfer LM, Winger G, et al: Large scale purification of butyrylcholinesterase from human plasma suitable for injection into monkeys; a potential new therapeutic for protection against cocaine and nerve agent toxicity. J Med Chem Biol Radiol Def 3:nihms5095, 2005

Mahoney JJ 3rd, Hawkins RY, De La Garza R 2nd, et al: Relationship between gender and psychotic symptoms in cocaine-dependent and methamphetamine-dependent participants. Gend Med 7:414–421, 2010

Mardikian PN, LaRowe SD, Hedden S, et al: An open-label trial of N-acetylcysteine for the treatment of cocaine dependence: a pilot study. Prog Neuropsychopharmacol Biol Psychiatry 31:389–394, 2007

Martell BA, Orson FM, Poling J, et al: Cocaine vaccine for the treatment of cocaine dependence in methadone-maintained patients: a randomized, double-blind, placebo-controlled efficacy trial. Arch Gen Psychiatry 66:1116–1123, 2009

Michels II, Stöver H, Gerlach R: Substitution treatment for opioid addicts in Germany. Harm Reduct J 4:5, 2007

Mravík V, Skaupová K, Orlíková B, et al: Use of gelatine capsules for application of methamphetamine: a new harm reduction approach. Int J Drug Policy Jan 15, 2011 [Epub ahead of print]

Newton TF, De La Garza R 2nd, Kalechstein AD, et al: Cocaine and methamphetamine produce different patterns of subjective and cardiovascular effects. Pharmacol Biochem Behav 82:90–97, 2005

Newton TF, De La Garza R 2nd, Grasing K: The angiotensin-converting enzyme inhibitor perindopril treatment alters cardiovascular and subjective effects of methamphetamine in humans. Psychiatry Res 179:96–100, 2010

Nordt C, Stohler R: Incidence of heroin use in Zurich, Switzerland: a treatment case register analysis. Lancet 367:1830–1834, 2006

Nordt C, Stohler R: Combined effects of law enforcement and substitution treatment on heroin mortality. Drug Alcohol Rev 29:540–545, 2010

Sekine Y, Ouchi Y, Sugihara G, et al: Methamphetamine causes microglial activation in the brains of human abusers. J Neurosci 28:5756–5761, 2008

Sofuoglu M: Cognitive enhancement as a pharmacotherapy target for stimulant addiction. Addiction 105:38–48, 2010

Sofuoglu M, Mooney M, Kosten T, et al: Minocycline attenuates subjective rewarding effects of dextroamphetamine in humans. Psychopharmacology (Berl) 213:61–68, 2011

Tanibuchi Y, Shimagami M, Fukami G, et al: A case of methamphetamine use disorder treated with the antibiotic drug minocycline. Gen Hosp Psychiatry 32:559.e1-3, 2010

Vocci FJ, Montoya ID: Psychological treatments for stimulant misuse, comparing and contrasting those for amphetamine dependence and those for cocaine dependence. Curr Opin Psychiatry 22:263–268, 2009

Volkow ND, Wang GJ, Hitzemann R, et al: Decreased cerebral response to inhibitory neurotransmission in alcoholics. Am J Psychiatry 150:417–422, 1993

Volkow ND, Wang G, Fowler JS, et al: Addiction: decreased reward sensitivity and increased expectation sensitivity conspire to overwhelm the brain's control circuit. Bioessays 32:748–755, 2010

Yahyavi-Firouz-Abadi N, See RE: Anti-relapse medications: preclinical models for drug addiction treatment. Pharmacol Ther 124:235–247, 2009

Zhang J, Malhotra AK: Pharmacogenetics and antipsychotics: therapeutic efficacy and side effects prediction. Expert Opin Drug Metabol Toxicol 7:9–37, 2011

Index

Page numbers printed in **boldface** type refer to tables or figures.